Volume 18

ADOPTION POLICY AND PRACTICE

ADOPTION POLICY AND PRACTICE

A Study

IRIS GOODACRE

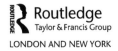

LONDON AND NEW YORK

First published in 1966 by George Allen & Unwin Ltd.

This edition first published in 2022
by Routledge
4 Park Square, Milton Park, Abingdon, Oxon OX14 4RN
605 Third Avenue, New York, NY 10017

Routledge is an imprint of the Taylor & Francis Group, an informa business

British Library Cataloguing in Publication Data
A catalogue record for this book is available from the British Library

ISBN: 978-1-03-203381-5 (Set)
ISBN: 978-1-00-321681-0 (Set) (ebk)
ISBN: 978-1-03-204965-6 (Volume 18) (hbk)
ISBN: 978-1-03-204970-0 (Volume 18) (pbk)
ISBN: 978-1-00-319539-9 (Volume 18) (ebk)

DOI: 10.4324/9781003195399

Publisher's Note
The publisher has gone to great lengths to ensure the quality of this reprint but points out that some imperfections in the original copies may be apparent.

Disclaimer
The publisher has made every effort to trace copyright holders and would welcome correspondence from those they have been unable to trace.

ADOPTION POLICY AND PRACTICE

A STUDY

BY

IRIS GOODACRE

with a Foreword by
ROBINA S. ADDIS

London

GEORGE ALLEN & UNWIN LTD
RUSKIN HOUSE MUSEUM STREET

PRINTED IN GREAT BRITAIN
in 12 point Fournier type
BY C. TINLING AND CO. LTD
LIVERPOOL, LONDON AND PRESCOT

FOREWORD

To adopt is 'to take (a person) into a relationship he did not previously occupy'. The picture of the homeless child adopted into the warmth and security of family life awakens a sympathetic response in each of us. Yet if the ideals called forth are to be realized we need to know a great deal about how and when to arrange adoptions and the best methods for selection and matching of child with adoptive parents. How much help if any should be available after the adoption is complete, is one of the most significant questions raised in Mrs Goodacre's book.

Further knowledge is also necessary about the subsequent history of the adopted child. This is largely an uncharted sea because once the adoption order is made there is no statutory provision for supervision or special help and it has been policy to treat the fact of adoption as confidential. It may be only by chance or in special circumstances, as when a child attends a child guidance clinic or appears before a juvenile court that his adoption is revealed. These stray revelations connected with maladjustment or delinquency give a distorted picture and we clearly need a view of an unselected series of adoptions, not merely of those which present a problem at some stage. Anxiety about interference in family life or breaking confidence have for long hindered social workers from making systematic enquiries but the necessity for such a study in order to improve adoption practice has become increasingly apparent. Not only Mrs Goodacre's success in winning co-operation from so large a proportion of the adopters approached but the wish expressed by many of them for further contact suggest that false fears had been built up and that adopters themselves welcome such an enquiry made with adequate safeguards and by the right person.

Here is an attempt to make a contribution to this necessary knowledge and this is believed to be the first book written by a social worker in this country who made a systematic study of certain stages of the adoption process and visited a random series of adoptive families (taken from the total list of adoption orders made in the selected area during a fixed period). A casework study was just the approach which the National Association for Mental Health had felt necessary and had advanced as long ago as 1954 when it published a Survey of Adoption Records.

A research study requires the right person to carry it out as well as the funds to support the work and both were forthcoming in 1960 when the Buttle Trust which, among its other interests, is concerned with the welfare of adopted children, gave a grant to the National Association for Mental Health to cover the three years study by Mrs Iris Goodacre. This generous action and the dauntless enthusiasm and skills of the research worker have produced this notable work.

Membership of the steering committee listed below indicates the professional interest aroused. It was believed that such a study would not only help social workers, and those directly concerned with adoption including adoption society and children's committee members as well as magistrates but it would also supply valuable material for teaching purposes. Adoption, since it highlights family relationship, is a useful field for all social workers to study. There are few casework records and little casework material available for the student or teacher, and many of our theories depend on untested assumptions about the ways in which people act and think and are not based on facts and personal interviews.

It is here that Mrs Goodacre makes her special contribution. In her talks with the adoptive parents and with the child care officers or adoption society staff her social work training and experience gave her a background of knowledge and made her sensitive to the implications of what went on in the interview. The disciplines of social work guide the selection of significant points from a bewildering mass of information and define the objectives of the visit.

A full case record of any one such interview with an adoptive parent might swamp the reader with fascinating irrelevances. Human nature and its expression in relationships (and here the special relationship of adoption is under scrutiny) has infinite possibilities and infinite attraction. If to avoid this dissipation of interest we attempt to use only selected points from case records, this again is a two-edged weapon as we are in danger of losing the dynamics of the situation, needing to know more in order to understand. This is the problem which faces all writers using case records.

Here it has been tackled by weaving actual comments made by adoptive parents and the social workers associated with them into the discussion of a particular attitude. It may seem like repetition to give the adopters' views of supervisory visits and then the social worker's own comments on her supervision but the discerning reader will see that the careful reviewing from different angles enables the whole to be seen in the round. The use of 'live' material makes it more vivid yet its restriction to apt quotation avoids the pitfalls of producing a human story which in its own right carries us away from the main argument.

The book has a serious purpose and with its special approach offers a rewarding study. It will appeal to many who have long demanded further studies and more information. Societies registered for adoption whether voluntary or as a function of the local authority and children's departments in taking up their responsibilities in adoption, have demonstrated a deep sense of responsibility and wish to promote research and increase understanding. The Adoption Act of 1963 specifically provides for research to be carried out. Many health visitors and general practitioners who have become interested in adoption, and take an active part in helping adoptive parents, share this anxiety for help in improving practice and would welcome a book such as this based on actual cases. Workers in the adoption field in general may be satisfied with the results of their work, but still be eager to enlarge their understanding.

The Buttle Trust is to be congratulated on its vision and generosity, the N.A.M.H. on its faithful sponsoring of the project through ups and downs and the National Institute for Social Work Training for grasping the opportunity to add this study to its important series on social work.

ROBINA S. ADDIS
February, 1966

ACKNOWLEDGEMENTS

THIS report was sponsored by the National Association for Mental Health with a grant from the Buttle Trust for Children, whose founder, the late Prebendary W. F. Buttle, was himself a pioneer worker in the cause of adoption. My thanks are therefore due first to the Buttle Trust for their generous financial support and interest, and then to the National Association for Mental Health for all the help they gave so freely.

Miss Robina S. Addis, O.B.E., was Chairman of the panel appointed to advise me. Her friendship, help, and constant encouragement, were invaluable. One conclusion to which her own adoption research led her —namely that a study should be made of all the adoptions arranged in one area—helped to shape the form of this project.

The other members of the panel to whom I should equally wish to express my most sincere thanks are Dame Eileen Younghusband, D.B.E., LL.D., J.P., representing the Buttle Trust; Professor David Donnison, B.A., J.P., London School of Economics; Dr Gordon Stewart Prince, F.R.C.P.I., D.P.M., Maudsley Hospital; and the Children's Officer (who, for reasons of confidentiality, must regrettably remain anonymous) who so generously offered the facilities on which the feasibility of the entire enquiry depended. The panel members' individual and combined contributions have left their mark on every phase and every stage of this report. The trouble they took and the time they gave make it impossible for me to thank them adequately.

I would also like to thank Mr William Strachan, Clerk of the Inner London Juvenile Courts, who kindly commented on legal aspects of the report.

It is to Dr Roy Parker of the London School of Economics that I feel so particularly grateful and indebted. Not only did he take on the onerous task of editing the report; he was responsible for transforming the mass of factual data into an orderly, clear and telling analysis. Directly, as well as indirectly, every chapter has been shaped and re-shaped by his efforts and his ideas. He did not spare himself in trying to ensure that better use was made of the findings.

I would also like to express personal thanks to each of the adoption agencies which gave me permission to pursue my enquiries. Their willingness to sacrifice time and their readiness to allow their aims and methods to be scrutinised was a spirited and generous gesture.

Equally indispensable to the comprehensiveness of the enquiry was the co-operation of the many adoptive parents who agreed to be interviewed. Their readiness to allow me to share their experiences and impressions made their accounts of absorbing interest, and more than compensated for the difficulties in completing the enquiry. If the help they gave so freely can be turned to good account so far as future adoptions are concerned, then this will perhaps be their true and enduring reward.

CONTENTS

1

INTRODUCTION

ADOPTION exists in various forms throughout the world and dates back to antiquity. Childlessness, the wish for an heir and compassion have each played their part in establishing it as an important social institution. Formerly it was often regarded as a means of furthering the interests of the adopters. More recently, in this country amongst others, the concept and purpose have changed. Attention now focuses primarily on the child: in principle, his needs, his right to love, security and a normal family upbringing are more clearly recognized. This has resulted from a greater awareness that children who have suffered the loss of their parents' care must be adequately compensated if their proper development is not to be jeopardized. In its turn this has led to more concern about how homeless and deprived children are cared for. Adoption is often seen as the most desirable provision if the child cannot be reunited with his own family. Indeed the Hurst Committee which reported in 1954 went so far as to claim that 'there can be no doubt that adoption is generally a much more satisfactory solution than any form of institutional care or even fostering'.[1]

The aims of English practice are adequately summarized in the following definition of adoption: it 'is the method provided by law of establishing the legal relationship of parent and child between persons not so related by birth, with the same mutual rights and obligations that exist between children and their natural parents'.[2] Ideally care is taken 'to protect the three parties

---

[1] Report of the Departmental Committee on the Adoption of Children, (Hurst) 1954, Cmd. 9248, p. 4. Subsequent references to this Report will be to the 'Hurst Report'.
[2] See *Standards for Adoption Service*, Child Welfare League of America, 1958, p. 1.

concerned—children, natural parents, and adopters—from risks which may lead to unhappiness'. Children for example 'must be protected from adoption by people who are unsuited to the responsibility of bringing them up or want children from the wrong motives'. Similarly, 'the natural parents must be protected from hurried or panic decisions to give up their children and from being persuaded to place them unsuitably'. In their turn the adopters 'must be protected from undertaking responsibilities for which they are not fitted or which they have not appreciated . . .'[1]

Adoption appears to be increasingly popular. The demand for babies exceeds supply and the number of agencies[2] concerned with the placement of children for adoption has grown. The importance of employing qualified child care staff is more widely recognized and in general measures which protect children awaiting adoption have been further refined. The legal disqualifications previously inherent in the adoptive relationship have been almost completely eliminated.

In spite of these changes, and the growing proportion of the population who are affected, remarkably little is known about adoption. Indeed practically no research has been undertaken. Questions that are crucial to the welfare of the child, the natural parents and the adopters remain unanswered.[3] The extent to which the protective aims of adoption are being promoted by agency policy and practice is unknown. In fact no serious assessment of the work of adoption organizations has been made. There is also an almost complete ignorance of the outcome of adoption and hence the consequences of granting orders (or refusing them) can only be surmised. Untested assumptions and popular theories abound. It seems to be widely believed for instance that privately arranged adoptions compare unfavourably with those sponsored by agencies, but that adoptions by relatives are satisfactory and straightforward. Systematic evidence for such claims does not really exist.

[1] Hurst Report, p. 4.
[2] Throughout the book the term 'agencies' is used to include adoption societies and local authority children's departments.
[3] See R. A. Parker, *The Basis for Research in Adoption*, Case Conference, September, 1963.

There are a number of explanations for the lack of research. In the first place, of course, the law endeavours to ensure that adoptive families shall not be at any disadvantage compared with naturally created families. As a result there is an inherent principle in legislation and practice that everything connected with adoption shall be treated as confidential. This has without doubt been a major obstacle to undertaking research, but although the privacy of adoptive families needs to be safeguarded, it is equally necessary to have sufficient knowledge to make responsible and appropriate decisions about adoption. It is impossible to gauge or improve the standard of service without knowing what happened as a result of previous decisions and procedures. It might well be argued that a real concern for the individual and individual family not merely justifies research, but makes it essential. The design of research can provide safeguards against breaches of confidentiality, as this study demonstrates.[1]

Another reason for the lack of research must also be mentioned. Neither the adoption societies nor the local authority children's departments, who might have sponsored such studies, have been in a particularly favourable position. It was not until the Children & Young Persons Act 1963 that local authorities were given formal permission to spend money on child care research. Most voluntary child care agencies have been and still are handicapped financially and the terms of their charters rarely permit funds to be diverted to research purposes. The shortage of staff has meant that few agencies have been able to undertake even minor research projects.

In any case research in this field is far from easy. Many organizations and individuals are involved and studies must be broadly based to include legal, administrative and welfare aspects. Consequently they are dependent on the close co-operation of several bodies and people who, between them, hold the key to the different sources of relevant information.

This enquiry was prompted by the general lack of research but particularly because of all social contracts except marriage, adoption probably has the most far-reaching consequences; and

---

[1] See also *A Code of Practice for Research in the Personal Social Services*, National Council of Social Service and National Institute for Social Work Training, 1965.

orders, which are irrevocable, are made when those most affected have least control over their destiny. In this study current adoption practices and the assumptions upon which they are based are examined with particular reference to the needs of the children and the adoptive familes. The research was limited to what happened in one particular area and entailed studying adoption organizations which placed children; how they worked, what assumptions they made and the problems they faced. It also required an analysis of the parts played by the local authority in supervision; the *guardians ad litem,* and the court at the time of the hearing. Equal emphasis was placed upon describing the reactions of adopters to their experience and on discovering what problems they were facing in the post-adoption period.

Although the design of this research had many advantages, it also had many forseeable limitations in addition to the overall parameters of time, money and confidentiality. In the first place it cannot be claimed that the results are typical of the rest of the country. For lack of published statistics there is no means of knowing how far any area is representative in the number of orders made or the type of placements. The Registrar-General's national statistics, for example, do not distinguish private adoptions from those which are agency-sponsored. Secondly, the method of selecting the adopters who were interviewed furthered the aim of making comparisons between various types of adoptions and it was not a random sample. The deliberate absence of any coercion in inviting adopters to participate in interviews will also have produced some bias: enquiry into the reasons for refusal was precluded. It must also be noted that adopters were visited once or twice only, and the impressions recorded were those obtained at one particular point in these families' lives. For reasons of confidentiality, no attempt was made to substantiate their accounts by reference to outsiders such as teachers or doctors. Furthermore, as only recently completed adoptions (i.e. orders made between 1955-1958) were studied, families containing older adopted children tended to be excluded.

The administrative boundaries of the area in which the study was made limited coverage to certain children's departments and adoption societies. Policy and methods varied as significantly between the two main types—statutory and voluntary—as between agencies of the same type. The particular agencies reviewed had a definite influence on the nature of the findings: the children's departments, for example, were regarded as specially fortunate (taking the country as a whole) in that staff complements were above average and a higher ratio of trained child care officers was employed than was usual elsewhere at that time. Thus, again, the findings could not be said to be truly representative. But this particular limitation can perhaps be turned to good account: for if the better endowed agencies offer scope for the development of their services, then surely the findings can be considered as of more than local interest.

Though every effort was made to ensure that the enquiry was comprehensive, natural parents were not interviewed, except in the case of mothers adopting their illegitimate child with their husband. This limitation was accepted because it was feared that adopters would refuse to participate if the writer re-established contact with their child's natural parents.

It also has to be borne in mind that because adoptions completed after 1958 were excluded, the study cannot claim to be a completely up-to-date record of practice. Various changes have occurred. For example, staff ratios in some agencies have improved; patterns of work have been altered, and in some cases policy has been modified.

The analysis was not undertaken from a legal viewpoint. Readers who wish to see a brief review of this aspect should consult Appendix 2. The book takes the form of a step-by-step account of the main stages in the adoption process, beginning with the selection of adopters and 'matching' the child, placement and supervision, and leading up to the hearing and the post-adoption period. At each point the work of the various organizations is discussed together with the reactions and impressions of the adopters. Separate chapters have been devoted to the particular problems of private adoption; mothers adopting their own children and adoption by other relatives.

The object of this survey was not merely to highlight what has been achieved. Equally it was to make a critical study of practice and the assumptions upon which it was based, and to indicate possible areas for the development of the services. It was also hoped that it would encourage a more informed public opinion about the three parties to adoption, as well as contributing to the training of those engaged in child welfare work. The promotion of more research which would further the interests of all who use the adoption services was another of its objectives.

2

SURVEY METHOD

THE practical possibility of this enquiry depended on finding a children's committee willing to allow the research worker access to the records which all children's departments must keep in respect of each child placed for adoption in their area. These are the most comprehensive records available: without such access it would have been extremely difficult to gain the important background information upon which many aspects of the study relied. One children's committee generously agreed to co-operate in this and several other ways. The actual area has nowhere been mentioned, for rightly, the committee was anxious to ensure that nothing should be written or said which might lead to any of the adoptive families concerned being identified.

The scope of the study is therefore limited to what happened in the administrative area of one children's department. It was further limited to the four years 1955-1958. These particular years were chosen to meet the challenge that the survey findings be relevant to current practice, yet not so recent that newly constituted adoptive families could be disturbed by becoming the subject of study. A span of four years was necessary to provide a sufficient number of adoptions of all types.

There were three main stages in the research. First the 295 case files pertaining to every order made in the area during the four year period were studied and as much information as possible extracted. Most of the statistics in subsequent chapters were derived from this source. The result of this examination showed that the orders could be divided into five major categories: those made to natural mothers and their husbands; those made to adopters who had had a child placed with them by a local authority;

those made to adopters who had proceeded with the help of a registered adoption society; those made to couples who had made private arrangements to secure their child (either directly with the natural mother or through a third party such as a general practitioner or matron); and finally orders granted to those who were adopting related children (for example, nieces, nephews or grandchildren). The numbers and proportions in each group are set out in Table 1 below.

TABLE I
The categories of adoption

	No.	%
I Adoption by natural mother and husband	102	35
II Adoption of children placed by a local authority	73	25
III Adoption of children placed by a registered adoption society	71	24
IV Adoptions arranged privately: either directly or by a third party	22	7
V Adoption by relatives	27	9
	295	**100**

Second, a study was made of the administration and policies of all the adoption agencies which had been responsible for placing any child in the sample. In all, there were fourteen organizations. Ten were registered adoption societies (two local, two regional and six national), the remainder were children's departments of which the host department was one.[1] Staff in each of these agencies were interviewed but most contact occurred with the staff of the host department. This was natural because it was their records which were being studied and it was they who undertook supervisory and *guardian ad litem*[2] duties in their area. Some adoption societies allowed certain of their records to be studied, but others were prohibited from doing so by their rules or constitution. Generally only one interview with representatives of each society

[1] Three children's departments had placed a number of children outside their boundaries and in this area.

[2] In adoption application courts appoint an agent, the *guardian ad litem*, to report to them and generally to protect the child's interests before the court (see Chapter 6). See Adoption Act, 1958, Section 9 (7) and Adoption Rules, 1959.

was arranged. The information collected from all the agencies reviewed, statutory and voluntary, covered a wide range but centred on three main areas: the agency's administrative organization; its service to natural parents, and its service to adoptive applicants. In addition some interviews took place with magistrates and court officers.

The third part of the study involved interviews with a group of adoptive parents selected from the 295 cases.[1] These took place from two to five years after the order had been made. The aim was to study adoption in the family context and to find out about adopters' experiences and impressions, particularly with regard to the actual process of adoption. One hundred families were originally chosen for interview, though for various reasons only 90 were actually seen.[2] The division of adoptions into the five categories listed in Table 1 either reflects the child's relationship to the applicants or the method by which he was placed. It highlights known differences in the organization and implementation of the adoption service and in the kind of problems which might arise. For this reason it was decided to select twenty families from each of these categories, so that the maximum comparative information could be collected. Within each of the five groups all families were ranked according to the day, month and year when the court granted their order and twenty selected at random intervals. The temptation to choose cases which according to the records looked particularly interesting, or where adopters might prove especially co-operative was thereby resisted.

To avoid any breach of confidence, the children's officer invited families selected for participation to state whether they were willing to be interviewed. These invitations[3] were delivered by hand to the adoptive father or mother by child care officers. By delivering letters personally to the addressees the risk that they might fall into the wrong hands was eliminated. Both the letter itself and the bearer reminded adopters that unless they

[1] Certain families were excluded before the selection.
  (a) Those known to have lived in H.M. service accommodation (7 cases).
  (b) Those known to have moved out of the area (12 cases).
  (c) In the case of mothers adopting their own child all adoptions occurring during a second or subsequent marriage (40 cases).
[2] See p. 24.
[3] A copy of these letters is provided in Appendix 1.

gave the children's officer written consent of their willingness to take part in the survey, the research worker would not be put in touch with them and they would hear nothing further. The voluntary aspect of participation was made absolutely clear. At the same time stress was laid on the fact that their co-operation would be of great benefit to future adopters and to all concerned with the welfare of adopted children.

This personal method of contacting adopters, and the presence of a professionally trained caseworker, familiar with the survey's aims and methods and able to answer questions and offer reassurance if necessary, no doubt contributed to the high response rate. This discreet method of introduction was appreciated by the adopters. Many said they enjoyed answering an appeal, and having the opportunity of participating in discussions which they felt were important and worthwhile.

Only small batches of letters were sent out at a time, to ensure that there was the minimum of delay once the research worker had received the invitation to call on the adopters in their home. When completing the consent-to-visit form, adopters were asked to name a day and time convenient to them. Where families stated that they did not wish to participate, they were replaced by the next one in that same category who had been granted an adoption order. The following table shows the readiness of the various categories of adopters to be interviewed.

TABLE 2
Response to survey invitation

	Accepted[1]	Refused
I Natural Mothers	17	10
II Local Authority adopters	20	1
III Adoption Society adopters	23	3
IV Private adopters	16	1
V Related adopters	14	3
	90	18

[1] That not exactly twenty were eventually chosen from each category is accounted for by several factors. In category I there had been so many refusals that the problem of getting the full quota began to require more time than was available. In category III some adopters had adopted more than one child in the period. In categories IV and V tracing addresses of those 'moved away' made it impossible to get a quota of twenty from the small number of adopters.

With the exception of mothers adopting their own child, where there were many refusals, it will be seen that the refusal rate was low. There were few discernible trends connected with refusal and rarely was there an indication from the files that this might be expected. In several instances mothers who had adopted their own child gave verbal consent when approached, subject to their husband's approval. Their subsequent refusal to take part suggested that in this group the adoptive father may have been the one responsible for the decision not to participate.

While a great deal of information was collected about the adopted child and the family as a whole, the principal focus of the discussions with adopters was their view of the adoption services. The interviewer had a clear idea of the areas she wished the discussion to cover, but no set order was followed: adopters were not asked to answer a series of specific questions. The interview technique employed was semi-structured. The topics which were of particular interest were indicated: such as when and how the adopters first arrived at the idea of adoption; how they set about locating a child; how they felt about going through the selection process and being supervised during the probationary period; what their feelings were about telling their child of his adoption and when and how this should be done. Many chose to give a complete chronological account of their experiences.

Although this method of collecting information has serious drawbacks (particularly from the point of view of recollecting and recording the mass of detailed material obtained), it also has overriding advantages. Because adopters were encouraged to take the initiative, points of particular significance to them emerged freely. The keynote of each interview was informality, so that each family could feel at liberty to reveal its individuality. If a formal approach had been employed, it is doubtful whether so much intimate information would have been made available. The opportunity adopters had of not merely giving information, but of exchanging views in the course of discussion was obviously appreciated and found stimulating. Perhaps in this way they may have been recompensed a little for the help they gave.

Because the creation of an informal atmosphere was considered essential the location of the interviews was never in doubt. The adopters' homes were most likely to sponsor confidence, candour and freedom of expression. Apart from the reassurance adopters had of being hosts on their own ground, home interviews offered the added advantage of causing them least inconvenience. Moreover, it made it likely that both adoptive parents would be seen. They were also free to arrange which other members of the family should be introduced to the research worker. In the privacy of their own home interviews went on undisturbed for as long as was suitable. Most adopters accepted the suggestion of an evening appointment. Almost invariably the subject of the visit—the child—was introduced and shown off with pride; many were specially kept up for the occasion. Once despatched to bed, the interview proper would begin. Generally this lasted for at least two and a half hours. Roughly half of the adopters were visited for a second time, and occasionally three visits were paid.

Thus in almost a third (90 out of 295) of the total survey sample, one or both of the adoptive parents was interviewed by the research worker. In most of these interviews (seventy-three per cent) both adoptive parents and the child were seen, although as already pointed out, the children left before serious discussion started.

The first part of every interview was devoted to a further full explanation of the survey aims, as outlined in the introductory letter.[1] Practical examples were given of the ways in which their contributions to the enquiry would be helpful: for instance, that child care officers often wondered how adopters really felt about being visited, and that they wanted to have suggestions about the timing and frequency of their visits; whether these should be by appointment and whether advice regarding telling the child he was adopted had been helpful. Secondly, adopters were told about the system of sample selection, showing why other adoptive families they might know would perhaps not be visited. They were reminded that though the research worker had been introduced by the children's officer, the survey was not connected with any local authority; they should therefore feel free to express opinions about the statutory services. Lastly, the two survey sponsors, the Buttle Trust and the National Association for

[1] See Appendix 1.

Mental Health, were always named and their interest in the project explained. By this time most adopters had overcome any initial shyness and could embark on the account of their own experiences.

Few adopters expressed much interest in these preliminary explanations. Only exceptionally did they put searching questions about the research worker's brief, or about the possible outcome of the survey, though many commented on the value of such an enquiry. There was, however, real curiosity about the findings collected so far: how other adopters had fared; whether they were encountering any special problems, and how they were being dealt with. A few adopters began by requesting that specific questions be put to them. Once launched however, only a small minority required prompting, though it was sometimes necessary to steer them towards particular topics. Unexpectedly little resistance was found to covering the whole field; more often there was too much to discuss and too little time in which to do it. No notes were taken during interviews; these were written up immediately afterwards. This was made easier in that the research worker already knew from the case file factual information regarding names, ages, placement agent and so forth.

What quality of response was obtained? There were, as might be expected a few disappointing visits; disappointing not because of adopters' unwillingness to help but because of apparently limited insight or observation, or, very occasionally, because they did not really participate freely. The great majority of adopters, however, were aware that their own and their child's position was a special one and that adoption had raised issues which were worth discussing. But many found it difficult to put into words their personal and emotional experiences. The most illuminating interviews were with the few really perceptive adopters who had not only found adoption a challenging and thought-provoking experience, but who were also able to express their own feelings and reflections easily.

3

SELECTION

In the inter-war years, the number of children in institutions, and the dearth of foster and adoptive homes meant that a couple's mere willingness to take a child went a long way towards warranting the acceptance of their offer. Agencies took pains to guarantee their children's suitability for placements: it was the era of 'blue-riband' babies. Today, however, both adoption societies and the local authorities receive more applications from prospective adopters than they have children to place. Even those couples who, out of a far greater number, are considered suitable usually have to 'wait their turn'. The selection process by which their suitability is decided is generally completed by adoption societies in two stages. The first usually occurs promptly, formally and often by post. It consists of the application of 'eligibility rules' and clearly has administrative value in that it does not require the attention of trained staff nor does it absorb much time. Limits may be imposed for instance on the basis of the applicant's religion, age, or the size and structure of their existing family. Rules such as these may reflect considerations which are thought to be important in safeguarding the child's interest, for instance the age of adopters. Other rules may serve an obvious rationing function, as when couples are rejected if they seek to adopt a third child.

Those applicants who satisfy the eligibility rules then go through a second stage of the selection process to determine their suitability as adoptive parents. In some instances these two stages are telescoped into one. Nonetheless the idea of these two stages, of assessing eligibility and then suitability, fairly represents what happens to most adoption society applicants. In the case of the children's departments who, at least in the survey area, had no fixed rules of eligibility, the applicants entered straight into the second stage.

Whatever the differences in the selection process, all the statutory and voluntary agencies concerned readily admitted that selection was not only their most important task, but by far the most difficult and time-consuming. They were agreed that no matter how carefully subsequent phases such as matching or supervision were carried out, selection was crucial to the whole undertaking and to the child's future happiness. The major danger, it has been claimed 'comes not in rejecting a couple who would have made good parents, which is often necessary if the ratio of applicants to children available is high, but in making a placement with a couple who would prove to be inadequate in fulfilling the adoptive parents' role'.[1]

The Eligibility Criteria

The most common rule related to religion. Only one of the ten adoption societies operating in the survey area would consider accepting applicants without a religion and then only exceptionally. Where societies had affiliation to certain denominations only applicants of a similar persuasion were usually accepted. Seven of the ten societies demanded that successful applicants should be practising members of their faith and church attendance was taken as evidence of this. Some societies were less concerned about denominational differences than with the more general issue of whether or not applicants were practising Christians. Without doubt however, to be a church-going Christian was a considerable advantage in negotiating the initial selection hurdle. To have no religion severely restricted the possibility of a successful application. Couples in this position might have been considered by one small local society or by the children's departments. The latter did not make church-going a condition of eligibility. But couples who professed no religion could find themselves at some dis-

[1] D. Brieland, *Selection of Adoptive Parents at Intake*, p. 1. Child Welfare League of America, 1959.

advantage, first because the majority of natural mothers had exercised their right to nominate the religious upbringing of their child and secondly, because of the insistence on the idea of religion which runs right through child care legislation.

It is interesting to see the national picture in regard to religious criteria and this is provided in Table 3 below which has been constructed from unpublished data collected in 1964 by the Standing Conference of Societies Registered for Adoption.[1] It covers 71 organizations in all. Eighty-five per cent of them will not accept applicants without some religion; seventy-five per cent will only consider Christians and fifty-nine per cent only accept church-goers.

TABLE 3

Adoption societies' policies on the religion of applicants
(National Situation)

	No Religion		Not Regular Churchgoers		Non-Christian		Couples of Mixed Faith	
	No.	%	No.	%	No.	%	No.	%
Will accept	5	7	25	35	11	15	47	66
Will *not* accept	60	85	42	59	53	75	12	17
Will accept exceptionally	1		–	–	3		5	
Applicants 'treated on merit'	3	8	–	–	1	10	4	17
Policy under review or no information	2		4	6	3		3	
	71	100	71	100	71	100	71	100

All but one of the adoption societies in the study area had rules about the age of adoptive parents. Eight of the ten had fixed an upper limit. For wives this ranged between 35 and 44 but was typically 40. Husbands were generally allowed to be a little older the limit rising in one case to 46. One society required adoptive mothers to be less than 40 years older than the child. The local authorities merely stipulated that applicants should be within the normal child-bearing ages. The national picture is again similar. Forty-five per cent of all the societies in the Standing Confer-

[1] Standing Conference of Societies Registered for Adoption, *Adoption Societies Practice*, Revised December, 1964.

ence's survey imposed an age limit of 40 for women. Sixty-eight
per cent of them had limits, between 40 and 45. This can be seen
from Table 4.

TABLE 4
Adoption societies' policies on the age of female applicants[1]
(National Situation)

Age Limit	No.	%
35–39	2	3
40	32	45
41–45	16	23
46–50	2	3
Less than 40 years older than the child	3	4
No fixed limit	12	17
No information	4	5
	71	100

In our local study four fifths of the adoptive mothers who had
been selected by agencies were between 25 and 40 when their
child was placed. None were over 50 and none less than 23.
Table 5 below sets out this information for the local authorities
and the adoption societies separately. Although the adoptive
mothers selected by local authorities tended to be younger than
those chosen by the societies, the difference is not statistically
significant.[2]

TABLE 5
Age of adoptive mothers at placement

	Local Authorities		Adoption Societies	
	No.	%	No.	%
20 and under 25	6	8	1	1
25 and under 30	23	31	16	23
30 and under 35	16	22	26	37
35 and under 40	18	25	17	24
40 and under 50	10	14	11	15
	73	100	71	100

[1] Compiled from S.C.S.R.A. data.
[2] Throughout, distributions are considered to be statistically significant when the
probability of their occuring by chance is less than 0.05.

It is of course difficult to judge how far any of these selection criteria seriously modified the pattern of applicants, for there is no information about the characteristics of those who were rejected. It may be, for instance, that in any case no one over 50 applied to become an adoptive parent.

The age of the selected adopters was also influenced by rules about how long couples must have been married before being accepted. An assumption, rather than a rule, was that they should have been married at least five years. This was not only claimed to offer some proof of infertility, but also of maturity and stability. Exceptions were made by certain agencies where a recently married couple had definite proof of sterility. The statistics however suggest this rule was fairly rigorously applied, for seventy-eight per cent of the agency-sponsored couples were known to have been married more than five years and only fifteen per cent less than two years. Table 6 below sets out this information. Once more, however, the effect of the rules may be less important in explaining this distribution than the fact that couples who apply to adoption agencies seem to take a long time coming to their decision.

TABLE 6
Numbers of years adopters had been married

	Local Authorities		Adoption Societies	
	No.	%	No.	%
Under 2 years	–	–	1	1
2 years–5 years	10	14	11	16
6 years–9 years	23	31	29	41
10 years or more	31	43	30	42
No information	9	12	–	–
	73	100	71	100

In some cases rules had also been made about marital status. Only one agency was prepared to consider a single person; and two would only consider widows exceptionally. Four societies however said they would not rule out divorcees, but none appeared amongst those in the survey. The children's departments were willing to consider widows, divorcees, and single people 'on their merits'. In contrast all the societies had some rules about one or more of these categories.

It has already been suggested by implication that infertility was to some extent also a criterion. The couple's health and their chances of having a child of their own were described as important initial selection factors by all the agencies. However, the degree of ill-health or the degree of uncertainty about fertility which would lead to rejection differed between agencies. Though most of them required a normal expectation of life, some rejected anyone who had suffered conditions such as epilepsy, tuberculosis, diabetes or mental illness.

Two societies accepted only childless couples in 'fairness' towards them, and because this policy was considered to be in the child's best interests.[1] Where this latter consideration predominated it appeared to be based on the fear of competition between 'own' and 'adopted' children and of parents giving preference to one rather than the other. Hence the choice of childless couples was not necessarily associated with rules about proof of infertility. None of the other societies nor the local authorities had any firm rules about existing family structure and size, though it seemed that some preference was given to the childless. The national situation was similar: nine tenths of the societies in the Standing Conference's survey said they would accept applicants who already had their own children.

The pattern which emerged partly as a result of the exercise of such rules and preferences (and partly it must be assumed from the type of couple who apply anyway) can be seen in Table 7. Sixty per cent of the couples selected by local authorities and adoption societies had no child already in their homes; and nearly twenty-one per cent of the agency sponsored families already had at least one other adopted child; in these latter families the proportion was higher (twenty-five per cent) amongst the adoption society cases than the local authority (sixteen per cent).

[1] See R. A. Parker *Decision in Child Care* (National Institute for Social Work Training Series, Allen & Unwin, 1966.) In this study the factor most detrimental to successful foster care was the presence of own children who were young or near the age of the foster child.

C

TABLE 7
The structure of adoptive families

	Local Authorities		Adoption Societies	
	No.	%	No.	%
No child in the home	42	58	42	59
One own child	11	15	9	13
Two or more own children	6	8	4	6
An adopted child	12	16	18*	25
No information	2	3	–	–
	73	100	71†	100

*Includes one family with three other adopted children.

†Double counting occurs for one family had one own and one adopted and another four own and one adopted.

These were some of the more common general stipulations, but it should be noted that rules were liable to be relaxed when a home was needed for a 'hard-to-place child'. In other ways, too, rules were not always as rigid as they might appear. Though all agencies enquired about a couple's chances of fertility, only thirty per cent of the records examined contained information that a specialist had been consulted.[1] Most societies in the survey contented themselves with a doctor's statement that conception was unlikely and three did not require any evidence of sterility or infertility at all. In this way several couples who had decided against fertility investigations had nonetheless been accepted.

The 'rules' discussed so far were in large part the expression of definite and acknowledged policies. It was considered valuable to see whether other patterns of selection appeared to be emerging which were either not appreciated by the agencies or not explicitly recognized. The social class of applicants might, it was felt, provide such an example. It is hazardous to draw any firm conclusion about the association of class and selection, for no information exists about those who were rejected. It is however possible to make comparisons between the two main types of agencies, local authorities and adoption societies, with somewhat more confidence.

---

[1] Nationally only thirty-eight per cent of societies in the Standing Conference survey demanded such evidence.

Table 8 below provides some interesting results and comparisons.

TABLE 8
Social class of adopters[1]

Registrar-General's Social Class	Local Authorities		Adoption Societies		All other adoptions		Census 1951[2] Survey Area	
	No.	%	No.	%	No.	%	No.	%
I Professional	3	4	14	20	9	6		4
II Intermediate	6	8	10	14	15	10		13
III Skilled	33	45	36	51	80	53		51
IV Partly skilled	26	36	5	7	31	21		19
V Unskilled	2	3	–	–	8	5		13
No information	3	4	6	8	8	5		–
	73	100	71	100	151	100		100

It can be seen that whereas only twelve per cent of adopters in the local authority group were in social classes I and II, nearly thirty-four per cent of those receiving children from adoption societies fell into these two upper classes. A surprisingly high proportion were in fact in social class I. At the other end of the scale thirty-eight per cent of the adopters selected by local authorities were in social classes IV and V, while only seven per cent of the adoption society couples fell into social class IV and none into social class V. This is a very significant difference. It may be that it accurately reflects the proportion from each social class applying to the respective agencies. This could be a reasonable suggestion, for most of the local authority adopters (ninety-two per cent) had previously been foster parents and we know from various studies of foster care[3] that foster parents are under-represented at both ends of the social scale. However, if upper class people do not become foster parents or more often approach the adoption societies, this too requires further explanation. This may be found in the claim of one local authority that it referred many upper class enquirers to adoption societies because it believed in the value of social background matching and had few children who would 'match' such applicants. Notwithstanding these provisos, the difference is so great that some part of it might

---

[1] See Registrar-General's *Classification of Occupations*, 1960.
[2] 1961 Census material on social class not yet available.
[3] E.g. P. Gray and E. Parr *Children in Care and the Recruitment of Foster Parents*, Social Survey, 1957; and R. A. Parker *Decision in Child Care*.

reasonably be accounted for by differences of selection policy. It is indeed interesting to find that no other factor so clearly distinguishes those adopters proceeding via the adoption societies from those who were selected by the local authorities.

Most agencies claimed to accept applicants from all walks of life: this may be true, but the partly-skilled and unskilled are under-represented and the professional and semi-professional groups over-represented, as can be seen from comparing the first two columns with the last in Table 8. One society did have the reputation amongst their fellows of employing something akin to a social and financial means test and was said to be perpetuating the concept of an élite of babies for an élite of applicants. However, for want of statistics about rejected couples there was no means of checking these allegations. It has often been assumed that adopters of lower social status were more likely to proceed privately than through an agency. In this study at least, as will be seen in Chapter 8, the evidence was quite the contrary.

From this analysis of the social class of the selected applicants there seems at least a *prima facie* case for assuming that this does operate to some degree as a selection criterion. This may not be something to be deplored. Indeed it may represent a genuine attempt to secure at least the material and financial well-being of the child.

Criteria of suitability

Once applicants had satisfied the more general selection requirements, some of which as we have seen reflected assumptions about suitability, agencies had the further problem of satisfying themselves that those they chose could satisfactorily fulfil the role of adoptive parents. Frequently they were more sure of the disqualifications. It was difficult to establish for instance whether 'ideal' parents were being sought or just 'average', typical parents. Most of the explanations about the final selection processes were difficult to reduce to concrete propositions.

However, the children's departments and the societies employing trained caseworkers were fairly specific about the criteria upon which they selected the most suitable applicants. Their views and the objectives of their selection interviews were similar.

They tried to satisfy themselves that applicants had good potential for adoptive parenthood by seeking to answer a number of questions. First they wanted to be satisfied that applicants were ready to embark upon adoption: that they had, for instance, sought advice about their infertility, that they had considered carefully what was involved in adoption and had had an opportunity to discuss this with a social worker. In addition it meant discovering not only whether their own needs could be met by adoption, but whether the child would be assured of a happy and secure upbringing, that the marriage was stable, and that material means were adequate. These agencies were also anxious to establish as far as possible, that applicants had come to terms with such problems as infertility and had faced the differences between 'own' and adopted children realistically. If there were other children already in the family, they felt adopters should have considered the repercussion upon them and should feel able to treat all their children impartially. While treating their adopted child as their own they should be able to admit to him that he was adopted. They should not be afraid of hereditary factors, yet be aware of their possible influence. In addition they should be able to help their child come to terms with his past, by neither keeping it from him nor by conveying a negative or judgemental attitude. This is a formidable list, unlikely to be completely satisfied and in any case difficult to translate into practical assessment. Nonetheless it gives a fair impression of the sort of qualities that these agencies claimed to be searching for in their 'suitable adopters'. Nothing so systematic or ambitious was suggested by the other agencies. It was more common for them to talk in terms of a 'flair for judgement'; or 'knowing by experience'.

SELECTION AND ORGANIZATION

Selection and selection policy both appear to have been profoundly influenced by the manner in which the agencies' work had been organized. For example, staffing, the role of case committees, the amount of delegation, the area covered and many other factors besides, all helped to determine the individual process and scope of selection.

Staffing and the problem of numbers

All societies employed some untrained workers at the time of the survey. Several had no qualified member of staff at all, though generally they were very experienced. The qualifications of the staff were apparently unrelated either to the number of years that the particular society had been in existence, or to the number of children being placed. The larger societies in particular were trying to recruit more qualified social workers and some ran their own training schemes. All the societies felt themselves handicapped financially, and they linked shortages of staff (and of trained staff in particular) with their shortage of funds and dependence on voluntary contributions. Some admitted their inability to attract and retain professional social workers because their own salaries compared unfavourably with those of local government social workers. This difference possibly helped to explain the fact that the children's departments in the area were fortunate so far as their complement of trained staff was concerned: as a result their selection of adopters was only undertaken by qualified staff. For the country as a whole, however, the situation amongst local authorities was by no means as favourable.

Staff shortage is a relative concept depending upon the amount of work to be done. During the survey period all the adoption agencies but one claimed to have many more applications from would-be adopters than babies available. One secretary said that they would take only one out of every four applicants. Two others estimated ratios of 1:12 and 1:20. Unfortunately there were no standardized methods of recording applications. Some agencies counted the total number of enquiries, others only those applicants who fell within the eligibility range or who were followed up. Hence comparisions are difficult.

Even when applicants who did not conform to the rules had been excluded, societies still found themselves with too many applicants. Further measures to reduce numbers had often been taken. For example applicants were deferred (possibly for months) before hearing anything further about their chances, or waiting lists were closed. One society maintained they could only investigate every tenth application. Another secretary said she automatically discarded 'unlikely looking couples' as, for instance, indicated by the style of their letters. Her annual report recorded approximately 8,000 applications received in the four years reviewed, but only some 400 babies placed. She had two administrative assistants and a part-time worker who was called in 'when necessary'.

The small proportion of couples selected for interview and the even smaller proportion accepted, made it surprising that several societies claimed that few really eligible couples were rejected for lack of a child to place with them. One explanation may be found in the system whereby couples applied to several societies simultaneously. Another, that agencies found it impossible to keep waiting lists up to date and hence strong and persistent candidates could jump their place in the queue. Thirdly, the precise meaning of 'really eligible' seems in some doubt.

The children's departments reported a rather different state of affairs. During the years under review they were not empowered to place children for adoption who were not in their care. They said they often turned away potentially suitable couples. The total volume of applicants and the ratio of those accepted and rejected were not easily discovered in their case either. Records were confusing since couples usually had to agree to 'foster with a view to adoption' and it was not always possible to distinguish between fostering and adoption applications. At that time the average case load carried by child care officers in the area was 70. The bulk of their work concerned boarding-out, approved school after care, and preventive work, and therefore the relatively few adoption enquiries received from any one area could be followed up without undue delay. Altogether the local authorities concerned placed between 20 and 30 children each year and estimated there were 150 adoption enquiries annually. This give a ratio of about 6:1.

Preliminary Enquiries and Interviews

Both to economize time and save couples from needless disappointment all the societies conducted some of their preliminary negotiations by post. In this way ineligible applicants were quickly identified. 'Only those who can fully and in every respect conform to the rules should pursue their application' was the heading on one of the forms currently in use. Again in the interests of economy, several societies used forms, stencilled letters and circulars.

For half of the adoption societies seen, one interview only was allowed for the assessment of those applicants who conformed to their rules. In these cases, there was little attempt to assess matters such as the couple's attitude to sterility, illegitimacy, or telling the child about his past. And as there were many practical matters to be dealt with during this interview, such as the next steps in procedure, no more than a superficial study of attitudes, personality, and general suitability could be made. Thus, for lack of time and perhaps of training, staff in these societies could not use the principle selection tools of a casework agency—namely the detailed observation of the relationship between the applicants, and between them and the social worker. Even societies that employed trained staff found that opportunities for preparing applicants for adoptive parenthood (as opposed to selecting them) were too limited. To a lesser extent this was also true of the childrend's departments.

Two societies emphasized the value of using two workers to investigate each offer—both in the applicants' interest and that of the staff. Responsibility was thereby shared, and it was claimed to be easier to avoid prejudiced assessments. One society arranged for both a male and female interviewer to conduct their enquiries, and where committees took an active part this was often considered to fulfil a similar function.

The local authorities' system of interviewing all couples who applied, and the vast majority in their own homes, imposed a big burden, though the number of applications they received was considerably smaller than the adoption societies. Their records confirmed that once the couple's apparent suitability had been established in a first interview, at least two further visits were generally paid before a final decision was reached. Continuity was the rule, only one worker undertaking the enquiries. Child care staff were supervised by a senior member of staff, and no decisions about acceptance were taken without reference to the children's officer. As all members of staff had a mixed case load they were able to invest a broad fund experience in their adoption work, although they had only undertaken a limited amount of this.

It appeared that the local authorities interviewed most of their applicants but seemed to reject or redirect about four-fifths of them. Adoption societies on the other hand received a far greater number of enquiries, selected a small proportion for interview, but having interviewed them accepted most. The character of the work done by each type of agency was therefore somewhat different.

By law, no child can be placed in a home by an adoption society until the premises have been inspected by or on behalf of the case committee. The wording of the regulations suggests a practical, factual enquiry, and the form issued by some societies for the use of the 'inspector' did indeed cover mainly factual aspects such as cleanliness, number of rooms and facilities. Certain centralized agencies saved time by using agents such as a minister's wife, and did not meet the couple in their home. The shortcomings of home inspections as distinct from home visits of a more intimate and extended kind were especially apparent.

Committee and Selection

By law, adoption agencies must place final responsibility for the selection of applicants in the hands of their case committee. The degree of influence exercised by the committee however varied considerably, as did their size and the role they played. Their composition also varied markedly. Some had almost entirely professional members whereas others were mostly lay people.

Some society committees were described as 'working', and by this was meant that they took an active part in vetting applicants, either by visiting their homes or seeing them before the committee. Other committees limited their function to the endorsement of their field workers' recommendations. As one secretary said: 'I can be sure that in ninety-nine cases out of a hundred, my committee agrees to my proposals'. In her case, verbal reports only were presented. Other committees decided nothing before making a detailed study of full written as well as verbal reports.

There was no more agreement amongst local authorities than amongst adoption societies on the interpretation of the committees' function. One local authority committee for instance, considered all applications in detail. Approval was no formal matter. The final decision was a joint one, taken by the committee in conjunction with the children's officer and the child care officer responsible for undertaking the investigations. Advance copies of records, notes and references, were circulated. Applicants were known only by number and very few cases were dealt with per session. A neighbouring committee limited itself to endorsing recommendations on selection. This committee thought that however well informed, they could never be in as good a position to judge as field staff who had met the applicants.

Area Organization

The size of the area they served aggravated the staff problems of most of the adoption societies: it also had a major influence on the charter of the work. Most of the well-known societies accepted applications from far and wide, even if they did not include the whole country in their territory. A few conducted their entire business from headquarters and delegated the statutory home inspection to a local representative. The societies that did not accept this limitation regretted the time lost in travelling. During the years of the survey adoption society workers were less generously supplied with private transport (and with other time-saving facilities, such as secretarial help) than were their local authority colleagues.

Most societies regretted that for want of time they could not offer a higher standard of service. This problem was exacerbated by lengthy journeys. As a result contacts with applicants tended to be limited and speedy; delays were inevitable and many aspects of selection had either to be telescoped, omitted, or delegated, regardless of avowed principles. As one example of the expedients resorted to, a society secretary described how, when visiting distant parts, staff accepted hospitality from one or other of the couples included in that particular selection round. The repercussions on the agency-applicant relationship may be questioned. Although another society was partly decentralized, its regional representative who covered the selected area was found to have cases scattered over several large county areas. The amount of overtime she and most of her colleagues accepted as normal (two or three evenings a week, often well into the night) was disturbing.

In contrast to most of the adoption societies, the children's departments operated in relatively small local government areas. In addition they allocated staff to a particular part of their area, so that the bulk of their visits took place within a limited radius of about thirty miles. All officers had cars and compared with the adoption society staff were well supported with office aids. The relatively small amount of time spent travelling permitted the staff to interview more applicants more often, more informally, and in more varied settings (in the office, at home, singly and as a family) than was possible for all but the two smallest local adoption societies. These latter shared the children's departments' awareness of the benefits of serving only a limited territory, easily accessible to staff and clients.

References

All agencies invariably took up references concerning the applicants' suitability. Most of the adoption societies did not indicate to the applicants the type of referees they would prefer to be nominated, but simply provided a space on their application form which the couple filled in as they thought best. The exception was that all societies prescribed that the applicants' doctor (and some that their minister) should also be nominated. Societies generally restricted themselves to postal references. As noted from the files, this system gave no guarantee that the referees were willing or able to commit themselves on paper on such a difficult matter as the applicants' suitability. There were variations in the amount of help given by societies to referees: some were admirably comprehensive and gave clear indications of what they most wished to know, others left everything to the referees' discretion. Some societies used sheets of paper only large enough to record brief answers to questions, such as 'Would you say that the applicants' home life was normal, happy and secure? Do you think they want to adopt for the child's benefit or their own? Do you think the child will have every chance to develop himself to the best advantage in their home?'

The local authorities on the other hand took up references

personally, and usually the child care officer responsible for investigating the applicants' offer discussed with them the persons they might consider nominating. Their only stipulation was that one referee should be the couple's doctor. However, children's departments sometimes took up medical references by 'phone (according to the records), and on this aspect were less well informed than the societies, all of which used a specially designed form for medical references. Not all agencies (whether statutory or voluntary) warned applicants that it was their practice to check with the police and with public health departments in addition to taking up references. If it seems proper to make these enquiries, it could be argued that applicants have the right to be so informed.

ADOPTERS' ACCOUNTS OF SELECTION

The Prelude

Many of those interviewed described the early part of their marriage and in doing so, made it clear that they had given little thought to the possibility of remaining childless or being unable to increase the number of their children. They had not reckoned with stillbirths, miscarriages[1] or infertility. Generally years had gone by before they were forced to conclude that their hopes were unlikely to be fulfilled. Indeed as pointed out already forty-two per cent of the agency-sponsored adopters had been married ten years or more when the child was placed, whilst only fifteen per cent of them had been married less than six years. Occasionally, an illness, accident, or operation, had suddenly blighted their chance of having children. But those whose hopes had dwindled slowly seemed no better fortified against their grief than those whose lot had been decided at one blow.

It will be remembered that seventy-eight per cent of the agency-sponsored adopters had no child of their own when they applied. Of those interviewed in these categories, eighty-four per cent were in this position. It was difficult to judge to what extent such couples had sought professional confirmation of their infertility, but amongst the childless couples interviewed one-

---

[1] Thirty per cent of the agency-sponsored couples interviewed said they had either a stillborn child or a miscarriage before they applied.

third had been advised that conception was either unlikely or inadvisable. Another third had learnt this as a result of undergoing full scale infertility investigations. A further quarter had either refused this course outright, or had been unwilling to complete the series of tests. 'We didn't believe in meddling with God's will.' 'We preferred not to know which of us was at fault.' 'My husband said he wouldn't have anybody messing about with me.' Again, these particular couples had few opportunities, according to their accounts, of discussing their attitude on this point with an informed adviser.

The majority of the interviewed couples, however, regarded medical investigations as desirable and necessary. They had not needed encouragement from others to find out whether their infertility could be remedied, but were glad to have done what they could to have children. As one remarked: 'It made me feel more reconciled to adoption.' Nevertheless, apart from the physical aspect, these investigations were invariably said to have been distressing and disturbing, and aggravated by lack of encouragement, explanation and continuity. A few had visited one specialist after another.

Comparatively little information was obtained from adoptive fathers about their reaction to finding themselves childless. It was usually through the wife that views about both partners' feelings were explained. Without exception the adoptive mothers were very forthcoming: many admitted that they were still not reconciled to their fate, irrespective of the happiness that adoption had brought. One mother, who was not unrepresentative, said: 'No one who has not experienced childlessness knows the desperate wish for a child; the deep, nagging, angry, endless pain; the longing to be pregnant; the emptiness; the jealousy of other people's happiness in their children; the feeling of unfairness and utter frustration.'

Depression and anxiety had been common to most of these mothers. One couple who could be given no organic reason for their childlessness and who were advised to 'live in hope', described how they exchanged their tenement for a caravan tucked away in the country. 'We spent our last penny on it. We'd been trying for a baby for ten years. We hoped that perhaps it would do the trick, away from it all. But stuck out there, living from month to month, we got more and more desperate and miserable.' Another mother said: 'I knew that I was made to have a large family, like all my brothers and sisters. Going to work was no help. We'd got everything, bar the one thing we wanted. There was nothing to work for, or to save for, or to look forward to. We'd sit solemnly at home, or take out other people's children. But it was so forlorn.'

Shyness and pride aggravated many a couple's sense of loss and made them still more vulnerable. 'At work they said, "Aren't you lucky: no kids, no nappies, and no mess." We didn't let on we were going through the tests, or about anything else. They could think what they liked.' One or two suspected angrily that their childlessness was ascribed by others to a fear of childbirth. Some added that perhaps they had been ready to see accusations or allegations where none had been intended. 'But at that time, just about everything seemed to get on top of you, and got you down.'

Diagnoses of infertility were infrequently available in the records and it did not prove possible to collect precise information about this in the interviews. However, it would seem probable that the knowledge or suspicion that one or other partner is infertile whilst the other is not may have repercussions on their relationship and upon their motivation for adoption. A few of the couples who had sought professional advice alleged that they had not been told which of them was infertile. The word most often used was 'blame', and there could be little doubt that knowing 'who was to blame' was something not easily dismissed. Adoptive mothers in particular seemed troubled by feelings about their own worth.

The Applicants' Attitudes to Adopting

Not unexpectedly perhaps, it was the wives who had generally initiated the idea of adoption. They seem to have been more sure than their husbands that life was incomplete without a child. Nevertheless there was nothing sudden about the decision. Many admitted that it had taken years to give the idea serious consideration. It was not simply that it had taken so long to establish the results of tests and treatment, though for many couples this had taken years. All the adopters seen had had some hesitation about the 'second-best' character of adoption, about their own suitability, and in general about the wisdom of this course of action.

Some couples said that each partner had been equally keen to proceed. However, there was much evidence to suggest that such unanimity (at any rate during the preliminary stages) had been the exception rather than the rule. 'I'll be frank about it: I swayed my husband to agreeing to adoption.' 'My husband saw me getting more and more depressed. My nerves were going to pieces. I got so that I couldn't go past a baby's outfitters without getting miserable. At last my husband gave in. He knew I was crazy for a child.' 'I saw the adverts for foster parents. I'd been watching the papers for weeks. In the end, I made my husband write away.' Some couples had remained undecided for months on end while one or other partner waited for encouragement from the other. Often, one partner's diffidence about ascertaining the other's wishes, and in judging how far it was wise to attempt to modify them, had prolonged the uncertainty.

Such accounts contrasted with the experiences of the couples interviewed whose decision to adopt had been associated with events such as stillbirth or miscarriage. Whereas agencies seemed uneasy about applicants motivated by the wish to replace a child, the adopters themselves appear to have had no such doubts. The situation of this group appeared somewhat different from that of the larger group who hovered for so long on the brink of decision. For the latter, two conscious decisions were involved: to become parents, and adoptive parents. The other wives had already been pregnant and they and their husbands had had time to adjust to this and the idea of parenthood. The experience might have reduced some of the apprehension and doubt about adoptive parenthood. They certainly seem to have come to the decision more quickly.

The Attitudes of Friends and Relatives

When they were first contemplating adoption few couples knew of other adopters. The opinions of relatives and friends had therefore counted for a great deal. Apparently, their views on adopting had usually been discouraging. Many adopters said that they had been warned of the foolhardiness of taking this step. 'Blood's thicker than water.' 'You don't know what you're taking on.' 'You don't know how the child will turn out.' These and similar warnings were familiar to most. The awe in which many prospective adopters were held when they broached the subject was not necessarily reassuring. The inference was, they felt, how lucky for the child, but how brave of you.

Adopters regretted that publicity seemed only to be given to undesirable cases. As few of them had been sure of the wisdom of adoption, the proverbial warnings made a considerable impression. The opposition of relatives had in particular caused much unhappiness. More disapproval was reported on the part of the adoptive father's relations than by the wife's. Possibly the seemingly closer bond between relatives on the maternal side had helped to foster greater understanding and acceptance of the adoptive mother's plans. Several adopters had ignored the forebodings of relatives. Others had postponed action, trying to reduce opposition and prejudice. 'Surely there's not going to be a bastard in *this* house,' exclaimed the mother-in-law of one young woman who had undergone a long series of fruitless operations. 'Why don't you try harder,' was one exhortation to a despairing couple, patiently trying to accept the gynaecologist's verdict that he could do no more for them. 'You're trying too hard, relax and forget about it' they were probably also advised, judging by the numbers who had had to contend with this particular piece of gratuitous advice. Most couples preferred not to confide in their relatives in the early stages; often it seemed because opposition was anticipated. Relations would only be told once the die was cast, maybe when a child had been definitely promised. 'It's our decision after all, and if they don't like the idea, that's their loss.'

In discussing the influence of others, apart from friends and relatives, several adopters felt they had received insufficient encouragement from either their doctor or their specialist. Some felt these could have played a more positive role in suggesting the idea of adoption and in drawing their attention to the available agencies. These comments were in keeping with the adopters' general impressions of that period: that on the whole those with whom they came in contact regarded adoption with suspicion and unfavourably. It is interesting to speculate how many more applications might be made if it were not for such a discouraging climate.

The Decision to apply for a child

Having decided to apply, couples began to anticipate adoption with excitement. On the other hand, they realized that their failure to achieve parenthood in the normal way would now be made public, as would many of their hopes and fears. They expected to have to prove themselves worthy of parenthood by physical tests and also examinations of a more searching and subtle kind. They felt they were placing themselves in the hands of officials over whom they could exercise little influence. Whereas other parents were only dependent on nature and on themselves, they had to submit to fallible and probably arbitrary institutions, and to the verdict of unknown persons. Nevertheless, despite all their doubts, they went ahead with their application to an agency, thus making their first positive move towards adoptive parenthood.

Their first practical problem was the seemingly hum-drum question of where to apply. This decision was far more important than most ever discovered. Even those with experience of adopting through different agencies were perhaps unaware that this initial choice not merely determined the standards of service, but also the likelihood of their obtaining a child. In fact chance was often responsible for their choice. Many said that they had been bewildered by the alternative roads to adoption. Not all were sure what the advantages were of agency-sponsored, as distinct from private adoption. Nor could they distinguish between the peculiarities of the numerous statutory and voluntary agencies. Admittedly some couples had little trouble on this score, particularly practising members of a religion. These tended to go directly to the agency associated with their church. A few couples had had to turn to friends or the advice columns of the press, or to the medical profession for help in locating an agency.

There was much criticism about this lack of publicity. In particular, adopters regretted they could not discover in advance the various agencies' individual rules and regulations. For want

D

of this information half of those interviewed had met with refusal from one or more agency because they could not satisfy particular rules about such things as age, duration of marriage, denomination, or the presence of 'own' children of the marriage. They could perhaps have been spared the need to apply again elsewhere if full information had been readily available.

It was not only the waste of time that made so many applicants regret these false starts. In whatever manner the refusal was made, whether or not reasons were given, and whether help in accepting the verdict had been proffered, the impression left on all but the most resilient was one of rejection. Where the lack of a suitable child had been given as the reason, few accepted this at its face value. Most of them concluded that rejection was a mark of their personal failure, and even at the time of the interviews, the sting was still evidently painful. However critical adopters were of the reason given for rejection and however much they considered it unjust, mistaken or irrelevant, the experience had in some degree undermined their confidence. Those whose contact with an agency had been purely impersonal were especially irate. 'They hadn't ever bothered to know us.' In contrast a few rejected couples had evidently been mollified by their agency's offer to discuss the matter. None had actually taken up this suggestion, but they felt less affronted, for their application had clearly been dealt with personally.

Multiple applications had been the rule either because couples had found themselves rejected, or because the waiting lists were closed or excessively long. By trying several agencies at once applicants hoped to proceed more quickly. 'The first society we tried warned us of a two-year wait. The second strongly advised us to change our mind and to take a boy, as the list for girls was so long. But the third found us our daughter in a matter of months.' It might be noted here that no adoption agency knew precisely how many of their applicants had also applied elsewhere, either before or concurrently.

Interviews

What were the adopters' reactions to their initial contact with their agency? Experiences and attitudes varied enormously. Some had been encouraged to 'hasten slowly'. Their agencies had provided interviews for the discussion of adoption in general and their application in particular. From the start, a personal contact had been established between these couples and one particular representative. All those seen by local authorities experienced this treatment. Apparently only a few of the adoption societies had dealt with applicants in a similar fashion.

Adopters applying to other societies had not found it by any means so easy to get started or to obtain an interview. Their enquiry and request was first dealt with by letter without the offer of an interview at that stage. Forms had to be completed and on the applicants' answers depended whether they would be seen. For them the opportunity of evaluating adoption itself had not often been provided and it was taken for granted that the couple knew what they wanted.

If less had been at stake, these latter adopters might have been less critical of this phase. As it was, their uncertainty about adoption, about their own suitability, and about their society's methods, were all heightened by the impersonal manner in which they had been dealt with. The difficulties of entering into correspondence on a matter of this nature, and the absence of the 'personal touch', had led to endless frustration. In particular reminders that their application was 'one amongst hundreds', and the receipt of cyclostyled letters and printed forms in response to their own intimate letters seemed to them to portray a lack of consideration.

Sooner or later however, all applicants in the survey had reached the stage of being interviewed. Common reactions included anxiety, mistrust, embarrassment, and also some hostility. 'We knew we had to put up with everything,' said one adopter quite cheerfully but with an edge to her voice. What, or rather how much, the agency would need to know had worried most of them. For a minority one interview alone had decided the issue. When applicants knew that only one interview was being offered they had felt particularly nervous. When they knew a series of interviews was planned their anxiety was somewhat less. The writer found that prolonged enquiries and repeated visits had been at least as acceptable as quick assessments. Indeed, the latter came in for criticism. 'It was a matter of answering questions and of cut and thrust.' 'You couldn't *talk* with her: she was checking on you, and you just had to try and answer properly.' 'It was formidable. I should say that being interviewed ought to have been more friendly and less formal. Then they could have had what they were probably after.' 'Had it been a child of mine that was being placed, I would have made a thousand times more sure about the home it went to. Only simple, straightforward questions were asked, which we'd answered on the form anyhow. There was nothing about what we were really like and how we got on.'

Most applicants had obviously been prepared to undergo thorough investigation. If this had not taken place, they felt rather surprised or cheated. For example one couple who had spent a long period searching their hearts not only about the advisability of adopting but also about their own suitability, was frankly dissatisfied with the service given by their adoption society. They were glad to have been successful, but had little respect for the obviously unqualified worker who accepted them after a brief interview.

Where only single interviews occurred there seems to have been an understandable tendency for these to be somewhat crisp and to the point. This not infrequently created a sense of antagonism in the adopters. 'We had a real grilling. My husband said the questions were impertinent. I felt our chances were nil when it was over. They seemed to doubt our relationship. And my husband made it plain that he wasn't going to discuss his pay prospects, as he didn't see what that had to do with it.' The right to demand answers to intimate questions still rankled where the relevance of these enquiries had not been made clear; where interviews had been too brief with little two-way discussion; and where the applicants did not feel that a personal relationship had been established with the agency representative.

In contrast, adopters who had been given to understand that careful and detailed discussions were as much a safeguard for them and their future happiness, as they were a safeguard for the child, often agreed that, 'They were very thorough indeed: but that was only right and proper.' About half of the adopters felt this way. Local authority applicants and a minority of those sponsored by a society said they had received a series of visits which had lasted anything up to two hours each. Generally, these couples (like those whose whole future hinged on one interview only) concentrated on making the impression they judged most favourable to the outcome. Being anxious not to spoil their chances, they had not felt really free to voice their doubts. But the opportunity to discuss adoption on several occasions was said to have been helpful though not easy. Many said they appreciated being treated as individuals, with their own rights and needs. In contrast those who were quickly 'vetted' seemed to feel that the agency's requirements had eclipsed their own needs and feelings.

Home Visits

All adopters recalled that at least one home visit, or 'inspection' as some called it, had been paid. This was found comprehensible and reassuring. They had been glad to show off what they had to offer. Many expressed a preference for discussing intimate matters in the security and privacy of their own home. At the same time quite a number subscribed to the view that 'it was difficult to show people your home when you didn't know exactly what it was they were looking for.' Where selection had involved a series of home visits applicants realized that it was they and not merely their material conditions which were the focus of interest.

The statutory home visit was not necessarily regarded in this light even by the agencies. This was confirmed by an adoption society worker who said: 'We consider these inspections to be the least important part of our enquiries. Homes are always so spic-and-span nowadays.' This society, which offered only one selection interview, employed a local agent to visit the home. This practice came in for occasional criticism. A few couples objected that they had had to divulge their private affairs to a local resident such as a vicar's or a doctor's wife.

Following the interview and the home visit, three adoption societies required their applicants to appear personally before the committee for final selection. Such interviews had usually been very brief and formal, and they too had served to heighten the couple's anxiety. Generally, these sessions had been devoted to giving advice—that the adopters should make use of infant welfare

centres, that the child should be given a proper religious upbringing, that he should be told of his adoption, and that the
applicants should let the agency know if they were worried.
Several couples felt that the strain of being interviewed by the
committee was offset by the likelihood that they would be accepted
having got so far.

There was no uniformity about the time that adopters had had
to wait between being interviewed and being told the outcome.
Where applicants had not been immediately rejected (as half had
been before), they had generally to count on a period of several
months before their own suitability was confirmed. Several
reported that they had been informed at the outset that no
decision would be available before a given period had elapsed,
but few had had the benefit of such a time-table. This waiting
period had been trying to most of the adopters, who reported
that their agency failed to maintain sufficient contact. This was
an even more common source of grievance in respect of the
interval between the time the applicants were approved and the
arrival of their child.

Adopters' summaries of this stage showed they were clear about
those points that were helpful in launching their application, as
well as about those which handicapped them. All agencies were
commended which acknowledged the applicants' right and need
for special consideration: efficiency, informality and speed, as
well as continuity of personal service ranked high for approval.
Adopters were particularly grateful where the ordeal of selection
had been lessened by having had full explanations of procedure
and several opportunities for the discussion of adoption generally.
All to some degree felt grateful to the agency that had selected
them and placed a child with them. But those applicants who
considered they had been dealt with somewhat impersonally
were more critical of their agency's methods, rules and staff. They
seemed to have been denied the reassurance which might have
helped them through this first phase. The sense of partnership,
election and support was absent as far as they were concerned.

4

MATCHING CHILD AND ADOPTER

THIS chapter considers some of the factors which influenced the all-important decision which child should go to which applicants. To some extent private adopters and those who adopt relatives can choose a child for themselves. Agency-sponsored adopters however (with whom this chapter is mainly concerned) are largely dependent upon officials. Their part is limited to accepting or rejecting a proposed infant, though they may be allowed or encouraged to specify the kind of child they hope to have. Hence it is important to clarify the basis upon which such crucial decisions are made. A most influential concept appears to be that of 'matching'. Ideally it is felt that adopters and child should be well matched. However, once this has been said it becomes difficult to discover *exactly* what this means or to reduce it to a series of practical propositions. What particular factors or considerations are thought to be good guides to successful matching and how far do these affect day-to-day practice?

AGENCY POLICY AND PRACTICE

None of the agencies reviewed, statutory or voluntary, was able to provide a formal policy statement on matching. Indeed they were less specific about this aspect of their work than any other. Not only did the importance attached to it vary between one agency and another, but the workers within the same agency were often divided in their interpretation of what 'matching' actually involved, and on the relative importance of the criteria which ought to be employed.

When trying to choose the 'right' child a few of the agencies seemed to rely in large part on the adopter's capacity to love any child because he became *theirs*. In effect, these agencies had only partially accepted the idea of deliberate matching. They depended more on the general selection of adopters, assuming that those chosen would make good adoptive parents to most children. The other agencies attempted to reinforce the adopter's parental instincts more positively by finding out what sort of child they wanted and then trying to match the child as closely as possible to these aspirations. But they claimed to aim at, and achieve, more than this: maintaining that the allocation of children was neither random nor merely a reflection of adopters' preferences.

There were few commonly acknowledged criteria, although religion seemed to be one. Even where the natural mothers had not exercised their right to specify their child's religious up-bringing, all the children in the sample had been placed in homes where the adopter's religion and that of the natural mother was the same, although not necessarily of the same denomination. Careful consideration was also claimed to be given by all agencies to the age and number of children the applicants already had. Generally the object was to place a child in the order that would have been achieved by nature. This was hardly a difficult task, however, since eighty per cent of the children placed by adoption societies and fifty per cent of those placed by local authorities were younger than six months at placement. For both types of agency together eighty-three per cent of the children involved were less than a year old when they went to their adopters. With few exceptions therefore children became either the only child or the youngest in the adopter's family. Indeed ninety-five per cent of the agency-sponsored placements fell into one or other of these categories.[1]

School and job attainments, as well as material circumstances, were said to be used as guides in narrowing down the choice of homes, for all agencies claimed to attach some importance to matching the social backgrounds of child and adopters. This aim was often frustrated, however, by lack of information about the natural parents (particularly about the fathers). Even when such

[1] Fifty-eight per cent of them became 'only' children; thirty-seven per cent the youngest. An additional proviso was made by one adoption society: that only 'hard-to-place' children (e.g. coloured, older or handicapped) would be placed with couples who already had two or more children, whether their own or adopted.

information was available the natural parents themselves were sometimes ill-matched in this respect.[1] Although no agency kept specific records about the social class of its applicants or of the parents of children needing homes, this could be assessed from occupational data. Tables 9 and 10 below compare the social class of the adopters with that of the natural mothers. They offer no evidence however (either for the adoption societies or the local authorities) that any close matching of child and adopters by social class was achieved. Indeed, the adopters in each class received children from mothers of the various classes in the proportions which might be expected had there been random allocation. For

TABLE 9

Social class of adopters[2] compared with the social class of the natural mothers in all placements made by local authorities

Social Class of Natural Mothers	Social class of Adopters									
	I and II		III		IV and V		No. info.		Total	
	No.	%	No.	%	No.	%	No.	%	No.	%
III	2	18	6	55	3	27	–	–	11	100
IV and V	2	7	15	54	10	36	1	3	28	100
Special categories[2]	2	9	7	32	11	50	2	9	22	100
No information	3	25	5	42	4	33	–	–	12	100
	9	12	33	45	28	36	3	7	73	100

TABLE 10

Social class of adopters compared with the social class af the natural mothers in all placements made by adoption societies

Social Class of Natural Mothers	Social Class of Adopters									
	I		II		III & IV		No info.		Total	
	No.	%	No.	%	No.	%	No.	%	No.	%
II and III	6	22	4	15	15	56	2	7	27	100
IV and V	7	20	4	12	20	59	3	9	34	100
Special categories[3]	–	–	1	–	–	–	–	–	1	–
No information	1	11	1	11	6	67	1	11	9	100
	14	20	10	14	41	58	6	8	71	100

[1] This might have been exaggerated by the tendency of unmarried mothers to ascribe high social status to putative fathers. They might, understandably, feel the child's adoption chances were in this way enhanced.

[2] Based upon Registrar-General's Classification.

[3] Included unclassifiable 'occupations' e.g. 'schoolgirl', 'housewife', 'mental hospital patient', etc.

instance, twenty per cent of the adoption society sponsored adopters fell into the Registrar-General's social class I. They adopted twenty-two per cent of the children available from social classes II and III and twenty-one per cent of those from social classes IV and V. If there had been a widespread policy of placing 'upper class' children with upper class adopters a more pronounced difference would have appeared.

Of course 'social background' matching is seen to have practical limitations when it is realized how restricted the possibilities really are. As a general rule, with both adoption societies and local authorities, the adopters were of a higher social class than the natural mothers. This may be due to many factors; to the nature of the demand on adoption organizations; to their selection policies, or to the range of alternative courses of action available to unmarried mothers. Whatever the explanation, the fact remains that in the cases where social class could be established sixty-two per cent of the natural mothers but only twenty-four per cent of adopters fell into social classes IV and V. On the other hand, whereas another twenty-four per cent of adopters were in social classes I and II a mere two per cent of natural mothers were similarly classified. It is not surprising therefore that in only thirty per cent of the placements where the social class of both parties could be judged was there precise matching. In most cases (fifty-three per cent of local authority placements and seventy-two per cent of the adoption society ones) the children were placed in a higher social class than that of their mothers. In only a small proportion (six per cent overall) was there a movement in the opposite direction. Since the local authorities had more (or had selected more) adopters from the lower social class ranges (forty per cent fell into classes IV and V) they had a somewhat better opportunity than the adoption societies to achieve social background matching.

Although this discussion is of interest as a backcloth to the claims which adoption organizations made about social background matching, the whole concept appears to require a more critical examination. In the first place if inherited traits or abilities are believed to be associated with social background then little is to be gained from making this a guide to matching unless information is available about the natural fathers as well as the mothers. In nearly a third of the cases agency-sponsored nothing definite could be discovered from the records about the occupation or social status of the natural fathers. Even relying upon apparently accurate information about the natural mothers may be hazardous, for in becoming pregnant and having an illegitimate child occupations may be changed; less skilled jobs may be taken temporarily. During this period therefore social class may appear to be lower than it is. The occupation of the father of the natural mother might, in these circumstances provide a more reliable guide to 'social background'.

If the environmental influences of social background upon children's development are also considered to be important, then this basis for matching must again be questioned. The great majority (eighty-three per cent) of children placed by organizations were less than a year old: many under six months. What influence is the mother's social class background likely to have had in this period, particularly when it is borne in mind that most children did not go direct from the mother to the adopters? In fact only twenty-six per cent of those placed by local authorities and thirty-eight per cent of those placed by adoption societies were direct placements. The majority of children had been cared for in the interval by someone other than the mother. Perhaps the social background of nursery staff, of foster parents or relatives ought also to be taken into account.

Thus whether social background is felt to reflect hereditary or environmental influences (or both), it is unlikely that most agencies have sufficient information to undertake such matching. However, the visible attempt to achieve this may be considered to have a reassuring effect on adopters and hence upon the ultimate success of the placement. This, as is pointed out later, certainly seemed important to many adopters.

In a somewhat similar vein, two agencies believed that interests and aptitudes ought to be matched. This again led to assumptions about hereditary and environmental forces which, so far as the writer knows, have not been substantiated. A third of the agencies also attached importance to matching of physique, colouring, and even likenesses of temperament. One society required that babies spent a period in their nursery so that information about temperament and appearance could be collected to supplement reports on the natural and adoptive parents. A lively, alert, active infant sucking lustily would, they felt suit a lively, active, enterprising young couple. Agencies which laid stress upon the importance of physical matching rarely mentioned the practical difficulties involved.

In view of the lack of any clearly stated or verifiable criteria for matching, two further factors were examined, although not specifically mentioned by the agencies. It was felt that there might have been an unrecognized tendency to match the age of the child and the age of the adoptive mothers (the younger women getting the younger children) and to match the age of the natural mother and the adoptive mother. The first possibility is again very limited, for although there was a wide distribution of adoptive mothers' ages (from the early 20s to late 40s) the ages of their adopted children were very tightly bunched under a year. For instance the vast majority of women dealt with by adoption societies, whatever their age, received a child under one year, and four out of five of them babies under six months. Local authorities dealt with a greater proportion of slightly older children and there was some tendency for them to go to the older applicants.

From the available evidence, there was no apparent policy on the part of local authorities or adoption societies to try to match natural and adoptive mother's ages. Of course since the median ages of local authority and voluntary societies' adoptive mothers were 32.3 years and 33.4 years respectively and only 22.5 years and 21.2 years for the natural mothers, it was unlikely that any exact matching could take place. None of the adoptive mothers was under twenty-three and only seven under twenty-five. In contrast two thirds of the natural mothers were under twenty-five and a third under twenty when their child was born. Even so, there was no significant evidence that children of older mothers were placed with older adoptive parents.

Thus there were few obvious explanations which helped to clarify the basis upon which children were placed by adoption agencies with particular adopters. It therefore seemed possible that other types of explanation might be sought, more implicit than explicit, and more connected with the actual work of the agencies than with 'policy' statements. For instance, it seemed that the numbers and categories of children accepted by the agencies had some bearing on the problem of 'matching'. The number of children placed annually by the organizations reviewed ranged from twenty-five to nearly five hundred. The 'type' of child they accepted and placed was largely determined by the criteria of 'eligibility'. Most societies, having a religious foundation, had strict rules about the beliefs of the applicants they could accept. These values, in turn, were linked with the denominational background of the children they placed. In this respect the local authorities and inter- or non-denominational societies had fewer restrictions. There were however, reasons other than religious ones which could make a child unacceptable to one agency (though not necessarily to another); these included:

(a) congenital abnormality;

(b) illness or accident to the child;

(c) his age;

(d) his legal status;

(e) a mixed or non-white racial origin;

(f) the possibility of inherited disease;

(g) a history of tuberculosis, epilepsy or venereal disease in the family;

(h) immorality or anti-social behaviour of either parent—such as incest, prostitution, or delinquency;

(j) the existence of several, or even one other, illegitimate siblings, and

(k) the absence of or insufficient information about the alleged father.

Certain adoption societies prided themselves on being highly selective in placing only 'guaranteed' babies from 'good, respectable homes'. Others (notably the children's departments and the societies that combined adoption with a general child welfare service) held that few, if any, children who were legally free for adoption should be ruled out as unacceptable. It should be noted that during the years under review (1955-1958) children's departments had no power to act as adoption agencies. Prior to the Adoption Act 1958, children's officers usually only accepted children who were both legally free for adoption and whose circumstances made it necessary for them to be received into care. If natural parents *would* not, rather than *could* not, care for their illegitimate child, they were referred on to one of the societies. This meant that many of the children available to local authority applicants had come from abnormal or unsatisfactory backgrounds.

Hence the numbers and types of children accepted for adoption played a part in defining the size and nature of the problem of matching. The problem was also influenced by the selection of applicants. If the initial criteria for selecting children and applicants were similar, then matching might not appear too difficult a task. If however, older, disturbed, or 'harder-to-place' children were accepted the need to select just the right home tended to be seen as more urgent. Since local authorities received a larger proportion of such children than the adoption societies, their greater emphasis upon this aspect of the adoptive process may be understandable. Similarly if an agency, by its selection policies, had recruited a very heterogeneous group of children or applicants (or both) not only was there more real scope for matching but the problem itself was considered to demand greater attention. Where initial selection was undertaken on the basis of certain fairly rigorous rules, the need for careful matching (and hence may be the need for trained and plentiful staff) could seem less pressing.

The discussion has touched upon the difficulty of placing disturbed or handicapped children, and this helps to show the misleading way in which the concept of 'matching' can be used. There was clearly no attempt, for instance, to 'match' a handicapped child with handicapped adopters. Nevertheless the term 'matching' is used about physical characteristics, social background and so forth. It is also used in a somewhat different sense for the process of assessing and taking account of the needs and capabilities of adopters and child, their strengths and weaknesses; in short their likely interaction.

Because of the range of their work certain agencies really could exercise effective choice in selecting a home for a particular child: others had less opportunity. The balance of applicants to children at any one time was clearly one important factor. How closely agencies could match depended not only on the number and type of children and applicants but also on the area covered by the agency; the number of staff it employed; their training; the time spent in getting to know the natural and adoptive parents, and the committee's roles in allocation decisions. The well-known national adoption societies covered a larger area, and accepted more children and applicants than either the children's departments or the regional societies. The latter felt themselves to be at a disadvantage when, for example, they had to find a suitable child for professionally qualified applicants requesting a baby whose parents were of a similar educational background. The small area covered by local authorities and regional agencies became an advantage, however, when the amount of staff contact with natural and adoptive parents was considered. In children's departments the same officer often knew both parties to the adoption, and even their immediate families as well. It was also possible to visit more intensively. This seemed to facilitate closer matching than was possible where (as in the case of the national societies reviewed) different staff dealt with natural mothers and applicants, or where the adoption staff had no personal contact with the natural parents beyond receiving their baby.

The ratio of staff to children placed also had a bearing on matching decisions. The secretaries of half the societies maintained that because of the pressure of work, no single placement, and no single aspect such as matching, could be allowed to take up an undue amount of time. Well-staffed agencies and those which only placed a limited number of children could, and did, spend much longer over each placement, both as regards collecting and imparting information. In contrast several of the most overburdened agencies had few or no qualified workers on the staff. Whether the less systematic matching methods noted in the case of the agencies employing untrained staff was due to the pressure of work, narrow patterns in the selection of children and adopters, or to the absence of training was uncertain. Untrained staff might be less able to elicit the information needed for matching and this could account for some of the differences in practice. Moreovetr, it might be expected that trained and untrained staff had divergent views on the necessity of spending time and resources on matching and on what this might entail.

A further barrier to matching was the system widely current amongst adoption societies of using agents (usually moral welfare workers) to interview the natural parents. A few societies accepted this as an expedient made necessary by staff shortages. Others felt it was no part of their function to deal with natural parents, beyond accepting their babies for placement. But whatever the reason for using agents, adoption societies said that this practice often prevented a close match. The shortage of moral welfare workers (particularly of trained ones), and their difficulty in establishing close contact with natural parents (especially the fathers), all had a bearing on the amount that the agencies ultimately learnt about the child's history.

It became clear that the case committees of adoption societies could also influence matching decisions. In some cases this was primarily a matter of pairing off the couple longest on the list with the child having the most urgent need for a home. It was unusual for committees to place the full onus on the field worker and merely endorse her recommendations. Several committees attempted matching in which cultural and social considerations played their part, as well as the wishes of the adoptive applicants.

In some of the smaller agencies which were without such facilities as reserved foster homes or nurseries, speed was often essential. The need to place babies quickly could take precedence over matching considerations because no real means of delaying or deferring decisions existed. The collection of adequate information and the choice of the 'right' adoptive home may both require time. In this respect children's departments and multi-purpose voluntary agencies were at an advantage.

THE APPLICANTS' REQUESTS
TO THEIR AGENCY ABOUT MATCHING

At the time their first child was chosen for them, most but not all agency-sponsored adopters said that they had put themselves more or less unreservedly into the hands of their agency. It had not occurred to some of them at that stage to formulate matching concepts. A few others had been prepared to accept the dictum (still professed by one of the societies reviewed) that 'to all intents and purposes, the child's natural parents are dead, so there is little point in delving into the past'. Only a very small minority of applicants did not express views about which child they wanted. These felt the needs of the child should be the overriding consideration. Thus, a few had been ready to accept children that did not 'fit', children of different racial origin, or children between the ages of the applicants' own children.

The great majority of adopters subscribed to the theory that the right choice of child was crucial to the outcome. Even so, probably as many as a fifth had accepted a child chosen almost entirely without their help, participation or foreknowledge. Many said they had done so because they were glad to try to emulate the ordinary parents' acceptance of their child. Their desire for parenthood was also important. Just as stipulations about the age or the sex of the child had been waived, so some had declared themselves ready to take the first child available. They often felt themselves to be in a weak position to make 'demands', particularly when they had had to wait a long time already. Occasionally their passive role stemmed from an appreciation of the burden imposed by choice—a burden which, because so much was at stake, some preferred their agency to shoulder. That the agency would know just which baby would be 'right' was a belief widely held. This seemed to reflect a considerable trust in professional competence which was often found to prevail whether or not close contact had in fact been established between the applicants and their agency. Where the same child care officer knew both the natural and the adoptive parents, her knowledge of both parties was another reason why some adopters had been content to leave matching mainly to their agency.

Most applicants had professed strong belief in the influence of environment at this stage. Repeatedly, they claimed that provided they were allowed to start with a really young baby they were sure to succeed in moulding him into their own pattern, and thus of assuring him, and themselves, of a happy future. However such views seemed to exist alongside concern about inheritable traits or predispositions.

In contrast to the 'passive' applicants there were a few who had

E

been very discriminating. They had demanded a considerable amount of background information about the child proposed for them and because of their belief in the overriding importance of certain factors (not all of which could be described as of hereditary significance) they had been exacting in their requirements. For example, some were insistent about nationality, even to the extent of differentiating between English, Irish, Welsh and Scots parentage. Evidence of the natural parents' high educational and occupational attainments were also important factors for a number of applicants. For a small minority a child's illegitimacy was a serious obstacle. Detailed information about the putative father and his family was demanded by others.

There were two points on which almost all agency-sponsored adopters had expressed some preference: namely, the child's age and sex. Except for a very small minority, the plea was for as young a baby as possible, preferably one straight from the maternity ward. In no case had subsequent events altered this widely-held view, that really early, speedy placement was crucial to a favourable outcome. Nearly two thirds of those seen who had had definite preference wanted a girl, though agency officials reported unaccountable swings in fashion. However, the writer learnt that once agency policy and the state of the waiting lists had been explained, numerous couples had been persuaded not to make stipulations about sex after all. As many as a third of those interviewed had accepted as their first child a baby of the opposite sex from the one initially requested.

Whereas requests for tiny babies suggested that applicants wanted to identify with 'ordinary' parents, their wish to choose which sex their child should be suggested that they would have liked to have availed themselves of this advantage over ordinary parents. Occasionally reasons were given to explain the preference; for instance, housing and the number of bedrooms. Yet many of those who had had a definite preference were at a loss to give a reason. Were some applicants afraid that promiscuity was a hereditary trait, and therefore that the adoption of a boy would be more prudent? Could choice and sterility have been linked— might there have been aversion to adopting a child of the same sex as the infertile partner? Occasionally, there was a hint that such considerations had played their part. The writer felt that they offered an important field for further investigation, although bearing in mind that many natural parents express similar preference and would probably also be lost for rational explanation.

This account would be incomplete without brief reference to the adopters' comments on the extent to which they were encouraged to state their views on matching. Some said that this topic had been fully discussed, but for numerous other couples it had been but one consideration amongst others, speedily and superficially dealt with. A few had feared they were in danger of being turned down altogether if they showed themselves to be 'too fussy'. At the same time however they all remembered being advised that if on seeing 'their' baby they had reservations, they should not hesitate to say so. Barely five per cent had taken advantage of this.

AGENCY POLICY ON INFORMING APPLICANTS ABOUT THEIR CHILD'S HISTORY

As with so many other policy matters, there was little agreement on how much information applicants should have about the child they were going to make theirs. A few societies divulged no more than the absolute minimum, and if any of their applicants preferred to know nothing, their request was granted. In contrast certain children's departments felt that applicants should be fully informed, and saw it as a mark of the couple's suitability that they shared this view. Somewhere between these extremes were the remaining agencies: they divulged *relevant* information. As relevance seemed to be subjective and as staff had considerable discretion, it was not easy to know just what was disclosed. Records were generally very inadequate in this respect, so that unless histories had been supplied by letter avowed policy could not be checked.

The placement of children with an adverse background highlighted the uncertainties which are surely basic to these differences in practice. The limited knowledge of genetics and the absence of follow-up studies of adopted children, both handicapped agencies in knowing how best to serve their applicants and the children. Not being certain what made a child suitable, nor just what information adopters found helpful or otherwise in rearing their child led some agencies to say little and others to divulge a great deal. But uncertainty was rife: even within an agency that believed in the importance of being frank staff disagreed as to how far potentially disturbing information should be made available. Such agencies were criticized by others for needlessly burdening the adopters (and ultimately the child) with anxiety. In their turn agencies that gave few details were criticized for not helping adopters towards a realistic, responsible outlook, and for storing up trouble for them later, when they had to tell the child of his adoption and try to answer his questions.

On what principles, then, did agencies say they were proceeding? Some supplied details to help adopters feel satisfied about the offer of a particular child, to arouse their interest and compassion and the desire to make him theirs. Some believed information to be essential if adopters were to bring up the child successfully, quite apart from their need for this information to answer their own, and later the child's questions. Surprisingly perhaps, the child's right to a knowledge of his background was rarely mentioned. Likewise, only one agency made specific reference to the natural parent's wishes: this agency said that mothers often requested that their child should some day know the circumstances leading to his adoption, so that he would know he had been relinquished for his own sake.

Seen negatively, agencies giving very full particulars could be described as protecting themselves against the sins of both omission and commission, particularly where frankness was used to encourage the adopters to decide their own and the child's suitability. In a similar fashion the agencies providing practically no information at all could be viewed as protecting themselves from subsequent criticism.

Practical considerations often played a part in determining what could and should be told. For instance one of the children in the sample was a foundling about whose background nothing was ever discovered; and several natural mothers alleged that the father might have been one of a number of acquaintances. One or two natural mothers refused to give details of the father; and where the natural and adoptive parents lived in the same area the conflicting rights and needs of the three parties also set a limit on the amount of information that it was felt could justifiably be supplied. But the most important variable was usually the amount of information the agencies themselves possessed. This depended upon the skill, time and care spent in eliciting it from the natural parents, which in turn depended upon staffing.

It was interesting to find that different agencies supplied the background detail to adopters at different times. Thus one society gave their adopters no information until after the child had been with them for some weeks: the applicant's love, it was felt, should be allowed to develop freely and unprejudiced. In contrast most of the agencies employing trained staff gave preliminary details before the applicants saw their child and then discussed the implications, enlarging on the information during visits after placement. Societies that did not offer more than sporadic post-placement visits could not provide their applicants with such opportunities and thus had no means of knowing whether the details met the adopters' needs, nor what construction they were putting on them. It could be said therefore, that whereas some agencies took trouble in finding out how far their applicants were willing and able to accept a particular child as their own, other agencies left much to chance in this respect.

THE ADOPTERS' VIEWS ON MATCHING AND ON THE INFORMATION THEIR AGENCY HAD GIVEN THEM ABOUT THE CHILD

Running through each interview were the adopters' comments on how their child had fitted in and, à propos of this, how they regarded their agency's matching policy. Of particular interest were their references to any points they had found helpful in integrating their child.

Those who felt able to identify with their child's natural parents said or implied that this had brought them closer to their child. Those who believed that his background had not been so very different from their own seemed to have found reassurance. The area of the unknown, and therefore the scope for anxiety appeared to be reduced. Specific details about the natural parents' age, appearance, job and interest were always prized and readily produced, as were any facts they had been given that were positive and socially acceptable. 'The father was a local footballer. The mother was said to be clever with her fingers.' 'The (natural) parents met in a youth orchestra. We're musical too, and the baby seems to be responding already.' The belief that interest and aptitudes might be inherited was common and was coupled with an equally widespread faith in environmental influences. Adopters seemed to have little difficulty in adapting themselves to a quadruple legacy.

Information that the child had been wanted by his natural parents was also valued. This too apparently helped the adopters' understanding, and made the natural parents more acceptable. Evidence of this kind was often thought to reflect beneficially on the child. 'We were told her mother was inconsolable when it came to the parting, and we've discovered the same depth of feeling in Janet.' That the layette had been exquisite, that one more report or a last photograph had been asked for, had all elicited sympathy and warmth. Adopters intended to pass such details on to the child to show him that he had not been rejected. Just occasionally, contrary information had stimulated the adopters' love. Thus one couple gloried in their child's waif-like, and impoverished state when he first arrived. It made them feel doubly needed.

Physical matching was of great importance to many. A large minority were convinced of a definite resemblance between themselves and their child, and the writer often had to concede that this was indeed the case. Luck must have accounted for many of the felicitous results achieved. 'Fair and slim, like all of us.' 'Just like my wife in temperament, and like me in build and colouring.' 'Exactly as I was, at his age.' One adoptive father said ruefully that he had often been accused of bringing home his wild oats: the resemblance between him and the boy was 'unbelievable'. Several children looked surprisingly like their non-related siblings. A few adopters also commented on the value to the child if he resembled them. He would be less often reminded of his status and therefore fewer explanations would be needed. However, even where no claim to physical matching could be made, likeness in expression, temperament, interest or turn of phrase were very widely claimed, with evident satisfaction. The adopters' views on the desirability of background matching were as might be expected. When first applying for a child, the importance attached to this aspect often corresponded with the applicants' own position on the social scale. Those who had themselves achieved something in life looked, in general, for promise of similar potential in their child, by reference to the natural parents' attainments. Some middle class applicants felt it was particularly important that the natural parents' educational attainments resembled their own. Yet some with few achievements had great ambition and amongst the successfully established some professed to be undemanding. There seemed to be a consolidation of opinion about the importance of social matching during the years that had followed placement. At the time of the survey interviews most of those seen were clearly ambitious for their child. By then, most adopters had devoted considerable thought to the part played by heredity and to what they had, or had not, been told about their child's past. Few any longer denied that hereditary as well as environmental factors were forces to be reckoned with.

The adopters' modified outlook was apparent not only from their comments to the writer, but in their description of the factors that counted when they applied for a second child, as nearly a third of those interviewed had done. By then, they had become more specific and more insistent in their matching requests. There was stress on the desirability of a good mental health background. At the same time adopters again returned to their earlier stand, insisting on their preference for a baby at the infant stage. Their greater insistence on their preferences at a second application might have been due to more experience and forethought; it might also have been accounted for by their 'stronger' position vis-à-vis the agency, in already having one child; or it might have reflected the tendency of some agencies to offer the harder-to-place children to established adopters.

The generally confident outlook of the adopters who were seen was notable, and many were gifted with a tolerant, and understanding attitude. Nevertheless, some were critical of certain aspects of their agency's matching or telling policy, and their

comments are important, even if criticisms were relatively in-
frequent or confined to details. A number of adopters felt that
because of their child's late placement there had been a bar to the
development of a really close relationship. As one adoptive
mother said: 'My son came aged ten days old, and from the start
I felt he might almost have been my own. But my daughter was
nearly four months old when placed, and we were bitterly dis-
appointed, having again particularly asked for a tiny baby. She
seemed "ready made" and she has never needed us as badly. Even
now she's independent in everything.' It was held that time not
shared with the child at this vital early stage could never be made
up. Some societies had a rule that no baby would be placed
before it was six weeks old and this was criticized by adopters,
who felt that though the mother could not consent to adoption
before her child was six weeks old, this should not prevent the
baby from being placed sooner.

The few adopters who had been told of a history of mental
illness or abnormality found it hard to conceal their anxiety. Some
dealt with their fears by trying to forget them. Thus two couples,
seemingly frank and open, failed to acknowledge that they knew
their child's mother to be mentally sub-normal, though the records
showed that the implications had often been discussed with them
during supervision. Potentially threatening details were sometimes reinterpreted by adopters, perhaps to make them more
acceptable. An ambitious semi-professional couple, whose child
came from a working class country background, was told the
natural mother had had a brain operation rendering her incapable.
The adopters' version to the writer was that the mother had
developed a brain tumour, the result of a kick while out hunting.
They, and many of the other adopters who were seen, needed
more help and guidance about the part played by heredity.
Equally, they needed further opportunities of discussing and
re-evaluating the information they had been given.

This need emerged clearly when illegitimacy was discussed.
Most adopters accepted that their child was the result of a lapse
from conventional standards of morality, and said with the
(sterile) adoptive mother, 'Where would the likes of us be, if it
weren't for the likes of them?' But it seemed that illegitimacy

nevertheless aroused real concern. Whilst stoutly defending their child against allegations which, they said, only concerned the natural parents, numerous adopters were nevertheless worried about the effect of illegitimacy on their child. Was there a connection between illegitimacy and a tendency towards promiscuity? Could it be hereditary, or was there a predisposition towards it? Even where adopters dismissed this idea, some were afraid that the disclosure of illegitimacy might precipitate their child into unmarried parenthood.

Another point which disturbed numerous local authority adopters was the knowledge that they and the natural parents lived in the same area. Even a distance of thirty to forty miles seemed to offer little protection from the fear of contact. Adopters who had received their child through one of the big national agencies were less afraid that the consequences of telling might ultimately cause the child to conduct his own enquiries into his origins. The few adopters with older children were particularly concerned on this question, and one or two had considered the advisability of moving right away.

All the adopters who had been told that their child was one of siblings had found this knowledge disturbing. They regretted having had some part in severing their child's right to connections which he might want maintained and were worried about how or whether this information should be imparted to the child.

As regards too little information, whether this was due to force of circumstances, to agency policy, or to the adopters' own original request, the outcome was to force adopters to realize increasingly the extent of their handicap. Without details on which to feed their imagination, the scope for speculation became uncomfortably wide. How would they be able to satisfy their child's curiosity? And how could those who chose to know nothing justify this attitude? One adoptive mother who had expressly made this request, so that there would be no need to lie or to hold back anything, strongly recommended that like-minded applicants should be protected against their own lack of experience. A small number of applicants who had been told that 'nothing was known about the father' pleaded that efforts must be made to obtain some details, both for their own sake and for their child's.

In the three cases where at the last moment a change of plan had led an agency to substitute one child for another, this had occasioned the greatest misgivings. The placing of a 'substitute' child emphasized so blatantly the hazards of adoption, and gave adopters even more scope to speculate on their fortunes. If others had known how often a child was placed without any comprehensive attempt at matching, they too might have indulged in more speculation than they did.

5

PLACEMENT

GENERAL CONSIDERATIONS

THE ways in which arrangements for the actual placement of
children had been made varied considerably. The full significance
of these variations becomes apparent when the differences in
selection and matching policies described earlier are recalled.
Casework agencies had spent time in getting to know their
applicants, in finding out what kind of child the applicants wanted,
and why. Societies that had telescoped their preparations for
adoptive parenthood into one or possibly two selection interviews
had given their applicants little chance to discuss their wishes;
nor had they necessarily provided them with information about
the child before they placed him. As one mother said, 'Our baby
almost seemed to drop into our lap'. Within four months of
applying a child had been supplied. Postal negotiations, one
selection interview and one home inspection by a local representative was the sum total of this couple's contact with their
agency. They then received a note that a 'suitable' child awaited
collection.

Most agencies saw their placement functions rather differently,
believing that as the initial preparations and contact could affect
the outcome the arrangements ought to be handled very carefully.
As far as possible the applicants were involved right from the
start. As soon as the agency had selected a child that seemed
potentially suitable and acceptable the applicants were given a
few details and were invited to ask for more information and to
visit if they wished. The accounts of the babies varied from those
giving little more than name, age, weight and appearance, to

others that were as comprehensive as they were sensitive to the applicants' (and the child's) needs. The following letter had been kept by one of the couples interviewed:

'Dear Mr and Mrs . . . . . .
     There is a three month old baby at present in our nursery at . . . . . . in whom we feel you may be interested. He now weighs 12 lbs., is in excellent health, has a mass of dark curls and seems to be a happy and lively little boy. He takes his feeds well, sleeps right through the night and seems in every way a good baby. His mother has been caring for him until recently. She is a tall, well turned out young woman of nineteen, who has worked as a clerk. She left school at fifteen, and qualified as a shorthand typist after attending night school for three years. She struck us as a pleasant person, who was obviously concerned to make the best plans for her baby. She said that she and the baby's father mutually decided that as they did not intend to get married, the baby had the best chance of happiness if he were adopted. The father is also nineteen. He served as an apprenticed mechanic until recently he joined the army. Though we did not see him, the mother gave us a photograph which shows that the baby has definitely inherited his father's good looks. We are told that the father was good with his hands, that his school reports were average, and that he was in his local football team. Both parents come from ordinary, good homes, and both, we feel, will be quite ready to confirm their consent to the adoption when the time comes.
     Please write and let us know whether you would like to know the name of the little boy, and whether you would like us to arrange your visit to the nursery. Miss . . . . . . whom you already know can then meet and give you all the other information you require.'

Most agencies preferred their applicants to see 'their' proposed baby at least once, regardless of distance. Since the national adoption societies generally had their nurseries, foster homes and applicants scattered over a vast area few of their adopters had been able to pay more than one 'preview' visit; and not many had had the chance of discussing with the agency's staff either the implications of the child's history, or their reactions to him between making his acquaintance and agreeing to his transfer to their home. The local authorites' and regional adoption societies' applicants were, on the other hand, better placed in this respect: most had had several preliminary opportunities of seeing and discussing 'their' child. Not only the proximity of the nurseries, but also the then widely current local authority system of 'fostering with a view to adoption' had sponsored a more leisurely pace during which a close link had been forged between child, applicants and child care officer.

The many favourable comments about the preview system testified to its value to adopters in helping them to adjust to parenthood and to integrate the new member of their family. Above all the meetings had given applicants a practical opportunity of confirming that they wanted to adopt and that the child selected was indeed the one for them. The opportunity to refuse the child if they so wished sometimes seemed to have given applicants the extra satisfaction of endorsing their agency's choice. Moreover, from many accounts, it often came as a shock when the adopters' first meeting with their child occured when placement was imminent. The strain seemed to have been more easily dealt with when first impressions and taking charge of the child had been separated by a short interval.

Previews had also been found valuable where, as in the case of a number of placements by local authorities, the child was no longer an infant. These older children had been visited repeatedly, taken out, and perhaps even invited for short stays prior to the final transfer. The benefits here were seen as mutual. In the case of anxious or inexperienced applicants too, opportunities to feed, bath and care for the young child had been greatly appreciated. One or two adopters without a knowledge of the rudiments of infant care had found it easier to admit this to nursery staff than to ask their more fortunate married friends for instruction. A further group of adopters, who were unanimous in their praise of previews, were those who had adopted a second child. At this stage applicants had evidently been more discriminating and perhaps cautious than appeared to have been the case when accepting the first child.

THE MEETING WITH THE CHILD

Most of the adopters who were offered a preview first saw the child that was to be theirs at a nursery. Usually, in looking back, they regarded this as a most suitable location because they had found themselves under tremendous strain and it had been helpful to be in the hands of staff who were used to dealing with this highly charged situation. Moreover, most said it had been reassuring to find the child was well cared for and nicely dressed. 'It would have made you feel that much more discouraged if you had felt *nobody* wanted him.' Occasionally though, nurseries were seen as baby marts. 'We've always thought back about those rows and rows of cots and the babies that would not be taken. The sight made us miserable and angry.'

Sad impressions were more often linked with visits to babies in hostels for unmarried mothers. Very few applicants had had this experience, but those who did had been acutely conscious of the mother's anguish, knowing that she would be anxiously awaiting their verdict. They had identified so closely with what they supposed were her feelings that their happiness had been marred. The fear of meeting the mother, or indeed any of the residents, had made it difficult to concentrate on the child they had come to see.

Two other locations for first meetings were foster homes and agency headquarters. The foster parents' tact had naturally gone some way to determine the smoothness of meetings but even so, applicants had been loth to display their feelings or their lack of experience. Some foster mothers were criticized: 'He wasn't much loved; he had a sore bottom. You could see they did it just for the money.' Other applicants were deeply moved and reassured by the foster parents' sorrow at parting with the baby. A few had gleaned additional information about the natural parents from the foster parents, but this had also caused some anxiety lest details about them might find their way back to the natural parents.

Where babies had been seen at agency offices, this was generally accepted by the adopters as logical and a few said it was useful to be able to say to their child later on, 'This was where you came from.' However there were adverse comments too, about bleak or official surroundings out of keeping with the applicants' mood. And again there had been fears of meeting the mother, who in some cases was known to have been waiting in an ante-room while the applicants were making up their minds. Guilt at depriving a mother of her child was more prevalent where meetings had taken place at hostels for unmarried mothers or at agency headquarters than at nurseries or foster homes where the parting between mother and child was known to have taken place already.

When recalling this first encounter, the intensity of the adopters' impressions often produced an apparent quickening of mood years after the actual event. Even if joyful anticipation had been the predominant spirit, courage and trust were equally essential. Most applicants had been intensely nervous about their own reactions and their partners'. Would they, could they, spontaneously and wholeheartedly take to the child?

It was usually the adoptive mother who described the day's events. Some compared the occasion with childbirth itself. Feelings of considerable elation, compassion and sadness had evidently been common. Though all were keyed up and very excited, not all found themselves as moved as they had expected: some felt incapable of demonstrating the full force of their emotions. Several said they had been afraid to give way in case they lost all control. Some recalled every detail vividly: the wait, the setting, the nurse, the child's expression as he was brought to them, while others remembered nothing except the point when they were handed 'their' baby. Although husband and wife had almost always been together when they received the child, not all agencies had specifically suggested this.

The child's helplessness and dependence and his need for parents did much to strengthen the applicants' courage. A surprising majority recalled that they had been able to respond with warmth straight away and had found ready conviction that the baby was 'theirs'. Others were more hesitant and discriminate. Several mothers seem to have had an image of the child they were expecting to find. 'I couldn't possibly have taken to just *any* baby: and I had to feel he was mine. I knew I'd just *know* if he was!' For most husbands this was above all their wife's day: if she gave her approval, then so would he. Possibly some of these fathers had not at that stage come to terms with the idea of adoption, for a number admitted that they had only been wholly convinced of the wisdom of the step long after placement.

Many adopters had attached significance to the child's reaction to them. Even where tiny babies were concerned, any sign that could be interpreted as favourable was invested with special significance. 'You see, he smiled, and we knew he loved us.' This woman had felt acutely conscious of robbing a mother of her child: she was overjoyed that 'her' baby had lain happy and contented in her arms. But the comment 'I could never have produced as lovely and perfect a baby myself' revealed something of the conflict of emotions aroused.

The importance of privacy was stressed. Adopters had wanted to give rein to their feelings without restraint, and wished to discuss their mutual reactions privately. Many had had a craving to strip their baby and to satisfy their curiosity about every detail relating to him. Above all, applicants wanted to establish contact with the child in their own way, undisturbed. Generally their needs were recognized by the agencies. It had been quite enough to contend with the turmoil of their emotions without the strain of having to be on guard before strangers. One applicant was particularly upset that a nurse removed the crying baby she so much wanted to comfort herself. She still remembered that she had neither gained the child's acceptance nor the nurse's approval. Another commented that she and her husband would have preferred not to have had to witness another couple's reactions: for both sets of applicants, they claimed, the day had been spoilt, for each was conscious of the other. It was interesting to see that the 'luck of the draw' featured in their particular account.

THE CHILD'S ARRIVAL

Looking back to the time of their child's arrival adopters also recalled their more general impressions. Some were newly made parents, whilst for others this had been their first opportunity to experience the differences between ordinary and adoptive parenthood. Their apprenticeship had not been without difficulty. While adapting to their new role, they were also having to establish themselves and their child in the eyes of their relatives and their community. Even if they felt able to see themselves as 'ordinary' parents, not all relations or friends had done so. Acceptance and explanations were demanded at a time when couples had not been sure how far their love was, or ever would be, comparable to that of ordinary parents. As one put it: 'We were having to defend our ideals when least equipped to do so.'

The physical and emotional changes of pregnancy often draw a woman closer to her family, particularly to her own relations. Forthcoming adoption did not always seem to act in the same way. Nearly three quarters of the couples said they had been reluctant to tell their relatives: they had delayed sharing approaching parenthood with them. In doing this, not only had they denied themselves practical help but also the initial moral support they often needed.

Where family bonds had stretched easily to encompass the new member the boost to the applicants' morale had been invaluable. But even where they had felt free to seek help and advice, most had needed time to overcome their inhibitions. One adoptive mother described her relief when her sister admitted that her child too sometimes seemed at first to be a total stranger. Her sister's chance remark made the adoptive mother's tentative feelings towards her newly placed baby more acceptable and allayed her secret feelings of guilt. As her store of confidence increased she found she could begin to enjoy her maternal status.

The writer's general impression was that where agencies invested time, energy, and skill in actively helping their applicants to prepare for the child's reception and integration the benefits were great. For the agency, there were further opportunities of preparing the adopters for their responsibilities and for assessing the effectiveness of their service. For the applicants a phased introduction provided the opportunity for committal and participation. In addition it offered a little extra time in which they could get used to their new commitments.

6

SUPERVISION

BEFORE an adoption order can be granted a child must live in the care of prospective adopters for a legal minimum of three months. Throughout this time they are supervised by the 'welfare authority' (i.e. the local children's department). Having once been notified, the children's department continues supervision until the order is made or until the child reaches the age of eighteen. Local authorities must by law supervise any child in their area awaiting adoption, including those placed by adoption societies.

The welfare supervision which a children's department undertakes must not be confused with the duties of the *guardian ad litem*. Guardians are appointed by the relevant court once the application for an order has been made. They are required to provide reports and in general safeguard the interests of the infant before the court. Their responsibilities include such things as ascertaining that consents to adoption have been given freely and finding out if any person not made a respondent wishes to be heard. The role of the guardian will be discussed more fully in the next chapter. It is mentioned here because misunderstanding can easily arise. In the study area (and many others) both juvenile and county courts appointed the children's officer as *guardian ad litem*.[1] These duties are in turn generally delegated to the child care officer who also has responsibility for the statutory welfare supervision of the child concerned. Hence one source of difficulty in discussing 'supervision' (and in being supervised) is the frequent

[1] This is not the practice however where the child concerned has been placed by the children's department: a neighbouring children's officer or probation officer may be nominated. It was not the practice in the selected area for probation officers to be appointed *guardian ad litem*.

performance of this and the guardian's duties by one and the same person.

This chapter is mainly concerned with the supervision of agency-sponsored adopters. The special position of related and private adopters is discussed elsewhere. Since only one adoption society undertook regular supervision it is the statutory work of the selected area's children's departments which is primarily considered.

SUPERVISION BY THE CHILDREN'S DEPARTMENT

In 1954, the Hurst Committee stated ... 'We think that it is now generally recognized that a waiting period, during which it can be seen whether a child will settle with the adopters, and whether they will accept him as wholeheartedly as they should if they are to assume parental responsibilities for him, is necessary in all ordinary cases.[1] They criticized local authorities 'which do not distinguish between the duties of welfare authority and *guardian ad litem* and begin at a very early stage of their advisory work to make enquiries which are the concern only of the *guardian ad litem*. Such confusion appears to arise from too wide an interpretation of their duties.'[2]

In discussing supervision the children's departments stressed the difficulties of interpreting the scope of these duties. Detailed regulations define their responsibilities towards foster children; for instance, the minimum frequency of visits is laid down. Where pending adoptions are concerned however, the only statutory guidance is that officers must 'satisfy themselves as to the well-being of such children' and 'must give such advice as to their care and maintenance' as appears to be needed.[3]

The child care staff who were interviewed challenged the Hurst Committee's view that the main significance of the three month period was to observe the mutual reactions of child and applicants. Outwardly at least most children were welcomed wholeheartedly, and almost without exception they appeared to settle well. In the staffs' opinion it was doubtful how far this initial adjustment had predictive value. They were equally critical of the adequacy of

[1] Hurst report, p. 15, para. 58.
[2] Hurst report, p. 16, para. 60.
[3] Adoption Act, 1958, section 38.

their legal directives. Rarely was the child's well-being in doubt, and only exceptionally did applicants require or request advice on 'care and maintenance'. If they did there was ample provision by doctors and health visitors, whose services were greatly appreciated: in particular, it was customary for adopters to reassure themselves about their child's condition by arranging for an examination by their family doctor within a short period of placement. Several adoption societies required their applicants to attend Maternity and Child Welfare clinics at least until the order was made.

Children's departments saw the purpose of supervision as twofold. First as a means of ensuring that the choice of home was in the best interests of the child's welfare; and second, as an opportunity of helping adopters deal with the social and emotional implications of their new role. They were concerned with problems which might occur in the family by virtue of the proposed adoption, and how best they could help the couple prepare to meet them. In most cases they felt it necessary to explore further how the adopters felt about their infertility; their view of illegitimacy; their attitudes towards their own or previously adopted children, and to telling the child about his natural parents and his adoption.

The staff felt that there were a number of obstacles to the discussion of such intimate matters. The first was the applicants' attitude to being supervised. The couple's experience in the pre-placement period was held to influence the kind of relationship that could be established during supervision. Applicants who were already familiar with casework methods usually appreciated the purpose of the discussions outlined above; they had encountered them during the selection process. But where, as in the case of a few adoption societies, selection and preparation had been cursory, the child care officers claimed it became harder to help applicants to put the supervisory period to constructive use.

Complications were also felt to arise from the local authorities' duty to supervise *all* pending adoptions. Certain societies, having undertaken selection and placement, then more or less severed their connections with applicants, leaving further visits to the welfare authorities. In such cases child care officers often found that they could not re-establish the degree of confidence and under-standing that had sprung up naturally between a couple and the society that had initially placed a child with them. One society continued to supervise regularly; others irregularly depending on the case. Even where strenuous attempts were made by adoption societies and local authorities to co-operate, the duplication that resulted in these cases was said to reduce the value of visits. The one society which did undertake regular supervision felt strongly that duplicate visiting, possibly reflecting different policies with regard to such questions as the provision of information, could lead to difficulties: difficulties in general of co-ordination and in particular of uncertainty on the part of adopters. Local authorities felt that the supervision of children placed by societies presented them with greater difficulties than the supervision of any of the other placement categories.

Adoption societies also had several different views about the welfare authorities' duties. Some queried the right of children's departments to share detailed information about a placement in advance of their appointment as *guardian ad litem*. Child care officers might, as a result, find themselves handicapped in helping the applicants for want of information about them or the child. Moreover at that stage applicants themselves did not necessarily know much about the natural parents or child's background. Adopters were often initially apprehensive of the local authority and this could be reinforced by being asked to divulge personal details all over again, having already 'laid themselves bare' to their society.

The actual amount of supervision appears to have been some-what limited as can be seen from Table 11. It is rather surprising to find that taking both these categories of adopters together, twenty-three per cent (thirty-three of one hundred and forty-four) had, according to the records, received no welfare super-vision visit. This may partly be explained by the confusion of guardian and supervision duties; but not entirely so, for in most cases the guardian is appointed some time after supervision begins. There is apparently another explanation of the higher proportion of local authority cases in which no record of a welfare supervision visit was found. Of the seventy-three

TABLE 11

Number of recorded home visits (excluding those classified as guardian ad litem) made by the local authorities

	Local Authority Placements		Adoption Society Placements	
	No.	%	No.	%
None	23	31	10	14
One or two	18	25	38	54
Three or four	16	22	20	28
Five and more	9	12	3	4
No information	7	10	–	–
	73	100	71	100

adoptions in this group only six (or about eighty per cent) of the adopters were not previously registered with their local authority as foster parents to the child they subsequently adopted: and all these six had been visited at least twice. Thus, all the twenty-three local authority cases without a recorded visit had previously been supervised as foster parents, often over many years. Table 12 below provides an indication of the extent to which the local authority adopters had already been acting as foster parents.

TABLE 12

Length of time children placed by local authorities had been previously fostered by their adopters

	No.	%
Under 6 months	11	15
6 months under 1 year	24	33
1 year under 2 years	19	26
2 years under 4 years	6	8
4 years or more	7	10
Not at all	6	8
	73	100

It seemed possible that those adopting for the first time would receive rather more attention from the supervisory authorities than those embarking upon a second or third. The tendency, however, although not statistically significant, was in the opposite direction. Those couples who had already adopted one child tended to be visited more frequently than those adopting for the first time. Taking all adopters in the study, three or more visits were paid to forty-four per cent of those couples adopting a second or subsequent child whereas only thirty-one per cent of those receiving their first child had as many visits.

It has already been pointed out that in both local authority and adoption society sponsored placements the children were generally very young. However taking *all* the adoptions in the sample it was possible to see whether the amount of supervision in any way corresponded to the age of the child. From Table 13 below it is plain that no such relationship existed.

TABLE 13

Child's age at placement and number of home visits: all adoptions

Child's age	Less than 3 visits		3 or more visits		No Information		Total	
	No.	%	No.	%	No.	%	No.	%
Under 12 months	106	61	62	36	5	3	173	100
1 yr.—under 5 yrs.	59	68	26	30	2	2	87	100
5 yrs. and over	23	68	10	29	1	3	34	100
No information	1	–	–	–	–	–	1	100
	189	64	98	33	8	3	295	100

There was, as might be expected, a clear and significant relationship between the number of visits and the length of the supervision period. This however was usually short; eighty-eight per cent of the children placed by societies and sixty-three per cent of those placed by children's departments were adopted less than six months after the applicants had notified the welfare authority of their intention to adopt. Most of the local authorities' adopters had previously acted as foster parents to their adopted child, and had been visited by child care officers over a period of months, or even years. In the case of the societies' applicants the situation was very different. With one exception adoption societies actively encouraged couples to proceed with their application from anything between one week and six weeks following the child's arrival. Here, child care officers felt that they had insufficient time to do all they would wish by way of supervision, particularly since there had been no previous contact.

Attention was also drawn to the size of the child care officers' case loads during the years in question. Responsibility for anything between seventy and eighty children was not unusual and duties included the reception of children to care, court and preventive work, finding foster homes, and supervising children in residential homes. Consequently home visits had to be limited in duration as well as frequency, even though it was often only during an extended visit that worthwhile levels of discussion were reached. These difficulties are reflected in Table 11, which shows that only a third of the agency-sponsored adopters received three or more visits during the supervisory period. They were also borne out by the brevity of many of the case records examined. These dealt mainly with factual matters and gave little indication of the impact of the child's arrival or the response to the supervisory service. In this they varied significantly from records on foster children in which emotional factors, assessments of relationships and so forth were a prominent feature and in which the child care officer's interpretation of her role as counsellor was much more apparent.

According to the staff, the real difficulty in supervision was not just a matter of time but also of timing. As they saw it, their visits coincided with a period neither conducive to achieving the aims of supervision, nor to establishing a close relationship with the applicants. Once adopters had received their child they were intent on identifying with 'ordinary' parents. They were inclined to reject the differences between biological and adoptive parenthood.[1] Such reactions were seen as understandable and indeed as valuable in helping the couple to come to terms more fully with the handicap of their infertility. Equally they were felt to place the parent-child relationship on a firm foundation. But in the staff's opinion these reactions also meant that applicants were not able to consider anything but the immediate situation. Indeed once their child had arrived adopters were said by the child care officers to see only as far ahead as the day of the court hearing. Despite all assurances, they lived in terror of the natural parent's consent being withdrawn at the last moment. Such concern was hardly

---

[1] See further H. David Kirk *Nonfecund People as Parents—Some Social and Psychological Considerations*. Fertility and Sterility, Volume 14 No. 3, May-June 1963.

conducive to discussions about ways of eventually representing the natural parents to the child. Likewise when new relationships were only just being formed in the family, discussions about own and adopted children were unlikely to be fruitful.

With the hearing imminent, supervision provided the last chance of drawing the adopters' attention to likely difficulties. The problem for the supervisor was to play both a reassuring role and yet to open the couples' eyes to the potentially difficult elements in the adoptive relationship. On the question of telling for example, all applicants were described as superficially receptive to the idea that adopted children should know early on of their adoptive status. Fundamentally though, many applicants were believed to be reluctant to face the full implications of telling. Knowing how much anxiety surrounded this topic, child care officers were unsure how far it ought to be pursued at this stage. Likewise they were also uncertain how far, in discussing other possible difficulties, they were providing adopters with cause for unnecessary worry and speculation. However, being aware that help would be less readily available to adopters after the order had been made, some felt themselves to be in the 'now or never' dilemma.

Several child care officers also expressed doubts as to their own personal competence to achieve something worthwhile through their supervisory visits. How far could they significantly modify deep-rooted problems such as feelings of inadequacy associated with infertility? Could they make any real contribution by extending the adopters' insight when contact was so very limited? Even where these personal doubts were not expressed, there was a widespread feeling of frustration about the difficulty of combining inspection with counselling. Several felt that the two roles were incompatible. How could the same officer be regarded as friend, adviser and confessor, when the applicants knew that a report on their suitability was being prepared upon which their chance of success might rest? Inevitably they would suppress some of their feelings about difficulties or drawbacks. Frequently the child care officers' explanation that their duty of verifying the adequacy of the child's care was not the only, or indeed, the main purpose of the visits, would be misconstrued.

From whichever view supervision was examined, the same questions seemed to recur. How could effective help be given at this particular stage in the time available, when applicants were least likely to accept it or understand its relevance?

THE ADOPTERS' VIEW OF SUPERVISION

Above all else the adopters were overjoyed to be entrusted with a child who would become their own in the forseeable future. This was the dominant impression of the period prior to the court hearing. They were pleased to share something of their sense of fulfilment, gratitude and pride with visiting social workers, especially since so many of them were able to report that their baby was making 'dramatic' progress. There was genuine appreciation of the interest taken in the child and many adopters also said that they had enjoyed visits from a purely social standpoint. Their relationship with the child care officer (and with the adoption society workers where they continued visiting) was almost always described as warm and friendly.

To varying degrees all recognized their dependence on officials, if only for the practical help provided in dealing with the legal formalities. Several had experienced the loneliness common to many parents of young children. This had been reinforced where they wanted to avoid the limelight, the inevitable questions, and the suspected criticism which adoption had brought in its train. In addition, those who had been reluctant to discuss their adoption with relatives or friends were also specially dependent on the outlet provided by supervisory visits.

Adopters readily acknowledged that supervision was 'only right and proper' and 'fair'. Agencies had to be certain that they had placed their children in good hands. 'We've all heard of cases where mistakes have been made; one can't be too careful where children are concerned.' The child's needs, and the agencies', were widely recognized. But having said they appreciated the necessity for supervision, adopters also made it clear that, as far as they were concerned, supervision had created much anxiety and sometimes even resentment. The necessity of having to prove their fitness as parents rankled, particularly as (at least retrospectively) the inspectorial aspect of supervision remained uppermost. Supervision was a symbol of the obstacles which lay between the applicants and their child. Many saw it as a trial period, in every sense: as a means to an end and a necessary condition to being granted the order. As a result adopters had felt reluctant to reveal their feelings to outsiders. They did not want to be disturbed in their endeavour to believe the child was almost theirs and were anyway not clear about the purpose of supervision. Hence they were constantly afraid that something they said or did might prevent the order from being granted.

Lack of confidence, misgivings and uncertainty about the rightness of the step they had taken featured in many accounts of the period before the court hearing. For many, the child's arrival had re-awakened strong feelings of longing and regret for an 'own' child. Others found it difficult to feel as wholly committed and involved as they had hoped, whilst some said they had been disturbed by the element of chance in the whole process. Couples appear to have been particularly introspective and self-examining during this period. As one mother said: 'For years I had longed for a child of our own. When that was not to be and Keith came I loved him dearly from the first. Yet I well remember how I used to panic, watching him lying in his cot looking at me. Had we taken on more than we could, or really *wanted* to cope with? Would we truly be able to love this particular child? Would we ever be able to stop asking ourselves whether we're just pretending he's ours—and will we always long he really had been ours?' Her husband's uncertainty had fanned her own doubts. She confessed that she had had qualms about proceeding because of the lack of his full support. Both partners had needed many months to feel convinced that the adoption had been right for them.

Thus applicants had not merely had to adjust to the inevitable demands of parenthood: over and above these there were the doubts and conflicting reactions. Ordinary problems seemed to acquire extra dimensions. Many found it equally difficult to judge how far their uncertainty and their mixed feelings were usual, comprehensible or permissible. At this stage some had probably been reluctant to admit their uneasiness or doubts even to themselves, far less to outsiders.

Some local authority adopters believed that there had been a subtle but unmistakable change in the authority's rôle once they became prospective adopters. Though feeling deeply indebted to them for having fulfilled their wish for a child, once the procedure was under way 'we were no longer sure which side they were on'. Nothing that came between the adopters and their child was tolerable. Comments such as 'visits always seemed to happen at the worst time' or that 'they came just to remind us he wasn't ours yet' indicated the degree to which applicants had felt threatened. Similarly, comments about 'surprise visits' suggested these were viewed with suspicion: bed-time or meal-time visits were sometimes believed to be deliberately timed spot checks.

Few adopters said they could recall having received an explanation of the local authority's supervisory aims and duties. This appeared to aggravate mistrust or misunderstanding. One adoptive mother still believed that the prolonged period of fostering required had been a testing device to assess her physical stamina. Two societies had rejected her on health grounds before the local authority agreed to place a child. The records show numerous discussions with these particular applicants advising them to delay on account of fears about the child's heredity, but this remained for them 'merely a blind'.

There was considerable criticism of the length of the supervisory period, particularly by the local authority adopters (see Table 12). Few had seen themselves in the distinct roles of foster parents and then as prospective adopters. Where delays had been advocated because there was concern about the child's potential for normal development, adopters protested that this was not justifiable. In their opinion adopters like 'ordinary' parents would not be induced to part with a child that had once been placed with them. Where delays were due to the natural parent's 'whims' in delaying consent there was even stronger criticism. Natural parents were held to have an unnecessarily long period of freedom in which to change their minds. It was they who were regarded as being the chief beneficiaries of the three month waiting period. It was apparent from these accounts that more time could usefully be spent by agencies in explaining their agency's function.

7

MAKING THE ORDER

THE climax is reached when the legal preliminaries have been completed by the *guardian ad litem* and all is set for the court hearing. On that day, if the order is made, the adopters assume all those parental rights and duties which would have been theirs had the child been born to them. It is valuable to see what happens on that day, what adopters felt about it, and what problems the court faced. Equally important is the preliminary work undertaken by the *guardian ad litem*.

THE ROLE OF THE LOCAL AUTHORITY AS 'GUARDIAN AD LITEM'

In the selected area it was the invariable practice of both county and juvenile courts to appoint the children's officer as *guardian ad litem*. It has been pointed out in the previous chapters that these duties were generally delegated to the particular child care officer already responsible for the statutory supervision of the child concerned. In cases where the children's department had itself placed the child a neighbouring authority was nominated, to ensure that the investigations undertaken on the court's behalf were truly independent.

Guardians must investigate all circumstances relevant to the proposed adoption and safeguard the interests of the infant before the court.[1] The guardians who were interviewed described these duties as 'no mean assignment', and two aspects in particular attracted a great deal of comment. First, they found it difficult to implement both the spirit and the letter of the law and second,

[1] The Adoption (Juvenile Court) Rules, 1959. Clause 8 and 9.

they faced certain difficulties in working closely with the courts that appointed them.

The guardian's principal responsibilities toward the respondents are to ascertain that consents to the adoption are given freely;[1] and, secondly, to find out whether any person not made a respondent wishes to be heard.[2] Interviews with natural parents taxed the guardian's competence to the utmost: rarely was any mother reconciled to the loss of her child. In such circumstances, to elicit piece by piece all the information needed to form an opinion on the mother's attitude and reason for consenting was frequently a painful process. Guardians said that in their experience it was unusual for mothers not to reaffirm their consent, and invariably they maintained that this consent was given freely and without pressure from other persons. However, guardians felt that they often had reason to doubt this: even if there was no pressure from other persons (which was difficult enough to establish) circumstances frequently seemed to force a mother's hand in parting with her child. For example, where support from her parents and the roof over her head were made conditional on her agreeing to part with the baby, could mother or guardian honestly submit that consent was freely given? Likewise husbands occasionally threatened wives with divorce unless they parted with the child which was not his.

Many guardians were concerned that mothers had not always had enough help or opportunity to consider fully the alternatives to adoption. They also felt that mothers were often ignorant of the services that did exist to help them, in particular about the advice the children's department could provide. Where a mother had not received advice from competent persons, doubts were inevitably raised as to whether the child was being needlessly deprived of his mother's care. This question was, of course, directly relevant to the guardian's duty to safeguard the interests of the child. But as they pointed out, by the time they arrived on the scene it was usually too late to offer such help, however much it might seem necessary. Moreover they were well aware there should be no suggestion that they had in any way influenced a

---

[1] Adoption Act, 1958. Section 4.
[2] The Adoption (Juvenile Court) Rules, 1959. Second Schedule. Clause 10.

respondent; their task was to ascertain,[1] not to counsel. In general they considered their work could be done with more confidence if provisions for unsupported mothers were extended and if the available sources of help were more widely publicized.

The guardian's duty to check that all who ought to be made respondents had been so named also caused occasional difficulties. The key person here was the child's mother. Some mothers concealed all information they were not bound to disclose— particularly the identity of their child's father. Where (as was usually the case) paternity had not been formally acknowledged, no affiliation order had been made, or there was no voluntary agreement by the natural father to contribute, he was not made a respondent. Consequently his views could not be ascertained by the guardian or by the court and it was conceivable that a mis-carriage of justice could result, because evidence that ought to have been given was not made available. Guardians were, of course, free to make representations to the court that a father should be made a respondent: but they were never certain when he might wish to be heard, or ought to be heard. Where adoption society placements were concerned, guardians felt that sometimes more effort should have been made to persuade mothers to reveal details about the father at the time they first sought the agency's help. If the opportunity was missed at that stage guardians were unlikely to be able to elicit this information when they arrived on the scene. Several guardians felt unsure about the natural fathers actual rights: they recommended that there should be further clarification of the law.[2] They were particularly burdened by the weight of their responsibilities *vis-à-vis* the respondents, whose rights they felt it difficult to safeguard. Whereas the other two parties to the adoption, namely applicants and child, appeared before the court, this was not usual in the case of respondents: consequently a particular responsibility fell on the guardian.

If a child is judged to be of an age to understand, then the

---

[1] The word 'ascertain' is specifically used in the second schedule of the 1959 Rules.

[2] Their confusion arose perhaps from the fact that although the natural father has a right to be heard in certain circumstances, he has not the right to withhold consent. The law appears to be that the natural father had not any right as such nor any pre-eminent position in obtaining custody, but he was a person entitled to special consideration because of the ties of blood. Lord Denning, M.R., in Re—o., AN INFANT (*Times* 31.1.63).

guardian must ascertain his wishes about the proposed adoption.[1] Most of the children in the sample were adopted in early childhood. Occasionally, however, where an older child was concerned records showed that the adopters had not shared the guardian's opinion that the child was of an age to understand. The crux of the matter here was that the applicants had not wanted to tell the child about his adoptive status and aimed at completing the proceedings without enlightening him. Guardians doubted how far children were in any case ever in a position to express independent views about their adoption. To that extent they felt that serving a notice of hearing on the child was a mere formality. In the guardian's opinion, the adoption of older children almost always reflected the existence of actual or potential difficulties that were not so apparent where young children were concerned. Though the adoption of older children occurred infrequently, when it did guardians felt particularly anxious about their responsibilities.

The largest measure of uncertainty and disagreement amongst guardians concerned their duties in relation to the applicants. How many visits ought to be paid before a guardian could properly claim that the child's interests were safeguarded? The records showed that usually only one visit had been made. How far could and should guardians explore to try to modify the applicants' views on the more fundamental issues that they considered relevant to the child's future welfare, such as the adoptive parents' attitude to his history, to his natural parents, to his illegitimate origin, to telling him he was adopted, and to mixed families of own and adopted children? Most guardians were convinced that unless they had combined their duties with welfare supervision it was simply not feasible to arrive at a worthwhile assessment on issues such as these. For by the time of their appointment the date of the hearing was fixed, and little time remained for the completion of their enquiries. In effect, the guardians seemed to doubt whether they could satisfactorily complete the task set them by the courts. Where their duties could not be anticipated by making a start on the enquiries during the supervisory period they felt that it was only possible to carry them out superficially,

[1] The Adoption (Juvenile Court) Rules, 1959. Second Schedule, Clause 3.

as best they could in the circumstances and in the time allowed. The guardian is required to submit a confidential report on each case and to attend the court hearing. The guardians were critical of their reports and considered them to be of limited value. They had little difficulty in presenting the factual background of the application. The Rules[1] prescribed exactly what items had to be included. But to the guardians this was only the groundwork for their investigation. They were concerned with the less tangible aspects too: the attitudes and feelings of applicants and child, the qualities of the relationship, and the capacity for adoptive parenthood. But despite their belief in the value of such information there was rarely any evidence to substantiate the formula which rounded off most of the guardian reports examined: namely . . . 'It appears that the making of the order would be in the interests of the infant.'

The guardians offered various explanations for this. First, the layout of the court reports then in use had been designed not by social workers but by the clerk of the council. Second, at that time (despite the Hurst Committee's recommendations and the legal directives)[2] a small number of courts in the selected area ruled that the contents of the guardian's confidential report had to be divulged to the applicants.[3] Either they were handed a copy, or else the whole report had to be read aloud at the hearing. Naturally, this made guardians exceedingly reluctant to include any personal comments that were not readily substantiated.

Even where it was not the court's practice to disclose the contents of the report, guardians admitted their reluctance to include their own opinions: they doubted the propriety of this and, indeed, one of the court clerks in the area had specifically discouraged guardians from 'telling the court what to do'. At the hearings guardians were always asked whether they had anything to add to their report. This was not the opportunity they sought however, for where they had doubts about the advisability of

---

[1] The Adoption (Juvenile, County and High Court) Rules, 1959.
[2] Hurst report, p. 87, para. 23 and the Rules Clause 9 (2).
[3] There is no legal authority for this view for '. . . parties have *no* right to see the confidential report, except in so far as the Justices or Judge think fit to disclose their contents at the hearing; they only have a duty to disclose the contents if the report makes allegations against a party on a matter relevant for him to deal with' re J. S. AN INFANT (1959) 3 ALL ER 856 AND A. G. (T. J.) (1963) 2 Q.B. 73.

G

making the order it was difficult to discuss this, or to comment, in the applicants' presence. Private meetings with the judge or magistrate, which guardians regarded as essential, were apparently exceptional. They were arranged only where this was specifically requested by the guardian, or where a legal or other complication had arisen; indeed it is doubtful whether this would be legal except on points of law. Guardians felt that, since their reports were an inadequate vehicle for conveying their views to the court, there was a definite need for a regular system of consultation. Without close co-operation they doubted whether the child's interests had always been as adequately safeguarded as the law intended them to be.

As the guardians pointed out, the system in operation in their area definitely favoured the development of a personal relationship between themselves and the courts, for members of staff each served a particular area. Potentially therefore, courts had the chance of getting to know their guardians well, and of appreciating the basis for their evaluations. Where advantage had been taken of this opportunity, they felt able to provide more relevant information upon which the court could make a decision. These courts also had the satisfaction of knowing that they had implemented not only the letter but also the spirit of the recent change in law, whereby, it is no longer permissible to nominate a corporate body (such as a local authority) to undertake guardian duties. A named individual has now to be appointed.[1]

THE ADOPTERS' VIEWS OF THE GUARDIAN ENQUIRIES AND THE COURT HEARING

The adopters had been only too anxious to set in train the arrangements necessary for making the child legally theirs. Prior to the hearing they had borne many of the responsibilities of parenthood without being entitled to the full rights. But although they wanted to see their plans fulfilled as quickly as possible, all admitted that this last lap had made them exeedingly anxious. Would the natural parent withdraw her consent at the eleventh hour? Would the court deem them unsuitable and refuse their application?

Recollections of the preliminaries included some mention of

[1] Adoption Act, 1958. Section 9 (7).

legal fees. Though very few agency-sponsored adopters had employed a solicitor, as many as a third of the others did. A minority of these wished to protect themselves from personal dealings with the respondents. In other cases where difficulties over consents had arisen, they had considered it worthwhile to have expert help. However, several complained to the writer that they had incurred legal fees (amounting in some cases to £30) unnecessarily. Too late they had discovered that the clerk to the court and the children's officer could, between them, supply much of the information and help needed. However, the various court clerks differed in their readiness to offer advice, and some applicants had already placed themselves in the hands of a solicitor before approaching their local authority. Attention was again drawn to the need to publicize further the work of the children's departments.

Though by law the choice of court clearly rests with the applicants,[1] both local authorities and adoption societies seem to steer applicants towards the type of court the agency preferred.[2] Thus some applicants had been told, 'county courts are more experienced' or 'judges, being legally qualified, can offer more certainty in difficult cases.'[3] These adopters virtually had had no option, for they felt they had to comply with their society's wishes. In rural areas, where magistrates and judges tended to be well-known local figures, some applicants had deplored this apparent lack of free choice. The fact that adoption societies seemed to prefer their applicants to proceed through county courts is reflected in Table 14.

Agency-sponsored adopters relied on their agency to see to the documents and, in particular, they had no responsibility with regard to obtaining the necessary consents. The other categories of adopters however, had no such help. Some who had had difficulty in obtaining consent, for example, complained to the writer that they had been delayed for months and sometimes

[1] Adoption Act, 1958. Section 9.
[2] The duplicated letter produced by one society says 'Please ask your county court registrar . . .' No mention is made of other courts.
[3] It is interesting to note the Hurst committee's comments in this respect: 'we were told that an impression exists in some areas in England that one court is "easier" than another . . . anything capable of giving rise to an idea that some courts are less careful than others is to be deprecated.' p. 22, para. 84.

TABLE 14

Type of court used[1]

| | Adoption Society Placements | | All others | |
	No.	%	No.	%
Juvenile Court	29	41	174	78
County Court	42	59	49	22
No information	–	–	1	–
	71	100	224	100

years. Some of these applicants criticized the local authority for tardiness or inefficiency, failing to appreciate their inability to become involved in this way. Having misunderstood their role in this respect, they had not been ready to credit the child care officers' other services of advice and supervision as having importance or relevance.

The serial number system[2] (an alternative to the use of names) was greatly appreciated by all the adopters seen. It gave them proof that their fears of becoming known to the natural parents were recognized and offered a degree of anonymity. Nonetheless, there was widespread criticism and concern that the forms sent to the respondents in connection with the hearing named the county or petty sessional division in which the applicants and child resided. They felt that this largely vitiated the benefit of serial numbers, particularly as petty sessional divisions tended to cover very small areas, which made the tracing of adopted children too easy. County courts had been preferred to juvenile courts by some for this reason. Criticism was also made of agencies that filled in the natural parents' addresses on the forms that had to be completed by the adoptive applicants. The latter said they did not want to have this information; and in any case felt natural parents were entitled to the same protection and privacy as adoptive patents.

As for the guardian's enquiries, most adopters remembered having been asked to verify their application forms. Several had

[1] Nationally in the same period about forty per cent of all orders were made in County or High Courts—thus the thirty per cent in the study area was rather less than might have been expected. No adoptions in the sample went to High Court.
[2] Adoption (Juvenile Court) Rules, 1959, clause 2.

been irked by the questioning to which they had again been exposed, and by the formality. Retrospectively the guardian's visit was often found to have fused with the adopters' recollection of statutory welfare visits. Though guardians will have endeavoured to convey that they were acting in the special capacity of court agent, few of the adopters seem to have understood this. Several had identified the guardian's findings with the verdict of the court, vesting all responsibility for the decision in the guardian. Though the guardian's report is of course directly relevant to the outcome of the case, the court alone is responsible for the decision. Misunderstanding on this point might have accounted for the general uneasiness about the guardian's enquiries and also for the view that the guardian was personally involved.

Practically all the adopters were critical of the courts; not only on the score of the adequacy of the accommodation, but chiefly because the setting seemed so completely out of keeping with their mission. In the selected area adoption hearings were always fitted in before the general business of the juvenile or county court. Adopters described how they, their child, other applicants and their children, guardians, agency representatives and legal advisers were all crowded together. In many instances the throng had been swelled by people awaiting the main court: adults and children, accused and defendants, witnesses, policemen and reporters. The lack of sufficient waiting rooms and particularly the absence of separate accommodation for parents with young children was regretted. Various adopters pointed out that the communal wait with other adopters invited comparisons: others objected to ushers who called out names in a penetrating voice. The public prelude to some extent annulled the aim of secrecy and anonymity and adopters regretted that 'their' day had had to be shared with so many others. Never more than half an hour had been set aside for adoption applications by courts in the selected area. Typically four or five couples found themselves summoned to appear at the same hour and within the next thirty minutes all would have been dealt with.

Most adopters had looked forward to the hearing as being the ceremony which symbolized fulfilment. It was the ardently awaited day when at last the child would be made theirs. Where judge or magistrate had appeared to recognize the adopters' happiness they were delighted. Whatever his reaction, they had clearly been impressed by what he said to them. It could generally be recalled years afterwards and had often proved to be a matter of pride and reassurance. For all of them, despite their qualms, the formal court hearing had marked the satisfactory conclusion to the whole sequence of events.

Most adopters, with the guardian's help, had had a fairly accurate idea of how the hearing would be conducted; despite this, almost all said they had found the experience an anticlimax, and disappointment coloured their accounts. They seemed to feel cheated of a long awaited moment of joy and of recognition. 'It was just a formality.' 'They didn't seem interested and they never looked at either of our children.' 'We were in and out before we realized it was all signed and sealed. The demand for a fee ("That'll be 12s. 6d. please"—as though it was a fine, but cheap at the price) and the clerk's curt dismissal made us wonder what they knew about it anyway.' Adopters like these were quick to point out the weakness of the system. Several regretted having to be 'arraigned against the law' and felt it was anomalous for adopters to have to appear in courts chiefly associated with the determination of guilt or innocence. Some who had experienced an impersonal or perfunctory reception suggested that applications might, with advantage, be transferred from ordinary courts to special tribunals. Many pressed for greater informality, particulary where (as happened in numerous instances) the formal court rooms had been used and not an ante-room. This recommendation reflects one made in 1921 which stated, 'We feel the importance . . . of keeping the sanction of agreements for adoption away from the atmosphere of criminal courts.[1]

PROBLEMS FACED BY THE COURTS

The history of legal adoption in this country is comparatively short, dating back to 1926. Even so, the list of contested High Court cases is long enough to illustrate the many legal and social considerations which can complicate the question of whether or

[1] Report of the Royal Commission (Hopkinson) 1921, Cmd. 1254.

not to grant an application. However, this section is not concerned with exceptional cases: it deals with the every-day problems which confront the courts whenever they try to ensure that 'the order if made will be for the welfare of the infant'.[1] Some of these problems are attributed to the courts by the writer as a result of her observations of court officials, child care staff and adoptive parents.

Dr McWhinnie points out, the Hurst Committee was ready to assert that 'if it is successful adoption is the most completely satisfactory method of providing a substitute home' while yet admitting that 'there is no statistical evidence of the percentage of happy results, but in the absence of evidence to the contrary, it is reasonable to suppose that the connection turns out well.'[2] The biggest difficulty for the courts seems to be that they work without the guidance which such knowledge of how past adoptions fared could provide. In altering the course of a child's destiny and in re-allocating parental rights, judges and magistrates are taking momentous decisions. But the outcome of past decisions, as well as present ones, remains unknown. Without this information, which systematic research could provide, confidence in these decisions must be based upon faith rather than evidence. Magistrates in particular may be especially conscious that they are working in the dark as they adjudicate in adoption cases: for in their capacity as juvenile court magistrates they are periodically confronted by evidence that 'the connection' may not have turned out so well where adopted children are charged with a delinquent act, brought before the court for non-attendance at school, or because it is alleged they require care, protection, or control.

According to the child care staff, certain courts had evolved a standard response to particular types of application. Thus some courts had the reputation of 'almost automatically' granting applications by mothers and step-fathers. Others were said to view with 'invariable distrust' applications by grandparents or by private adopters. As yet, there is little evidence that one

---

[1] Adoption Act, 1958, Section 7 (b).
[2] A. M. McWhinnie, 'A Study of Adoption—the social circumstances and adjustment in adult life of 58 adopted children.' (Phd. thesis, Edinburgh University, 1959) Unpublished. Citation from Report of the Care of Children Committee (Curtis) 1946. Cmd. 6922, p. 148, para 448.

particular category of adopters or children can be assumed to be more successful than another. Research could help to dispel prejudice and provide practical guidance.

The child care staff also expressed concern about the different character of the adoption proceedings in the various courts which they attended. The writer confirmed this impression, and ascribed it mainly to differences of role, personality, training, and qualification of the magistrates or judges and in some cases of the court clerk. At the time of the enquiry, county court judges and magistrates in the selected area had no established system of exchanging information about adoption proceedings. There were no organized opportunities for magistrates to observe the work of their colleagues on other benches. Indeed such exchanges or visits of observation would be out of order because adoption proceedings must be held *in camera*. Training was not compulsory for magistrates, although it is proposed that it shall become so for those newly appointed. But as adoption concerns only justices serving in juvenile courts, and as adoption cases account for only a small fraction of the time spent on court business, it is unlikely that training courses for magistrates will devote much attention to this subject. Some of the courts reviewed dealt with very few adoptions and hence their store of experience could only slowly be enlarged. Consequently, the need to make further use of local opportunities to exchange views and information was all the more apparent.

But even were opportunities for such exchanges plentiful, and magistrates trained and experienced in this work, not all difficulties could be overcome. It has been claimed that 'no colour should be given to the impression that the court acts as a rubber stamp for giving effect to the views of the guardian ... responsibility for making or refusing an order rests upon the court'.[1] In spite of this, the courts did appear to rely heavily on their guardians' reports and will presumably continue to do so. Except where interim orders are made, courts see applicants and child on one occasion only and under highly artificial conditions. The court can usually satisfy itself with little difficulty about the legal aspects of the case. But since adoption is not merely a legal contract but

[1] Hurst committee, p. 23, para. 86.

one in which social and emotional considerations are of prime importance, the inevitable question arises: can courts as now constituted really claim to be in a position to decide whether the order promotes the child's interests? Are courts in fact competent to do more than endorse the opinions and impressions of the welfare authority and guardian?

The courts in the selected area allowed the barest minimum of time for dealing with applicants. Apparently therefore their interpretation of their function in discharging their responsibilities differed from the Hurst Committee's ideas. Shortage of time was perhaps a matter of necessity not of choice. But the writer felt that the speed of despatch (normally between five and ten minutes) clearly indicated that courts preferred to consider cases on principle and not as individuals. Otherwise arrangements would have been different, a little more time would have been allotted to each application, and the fuller implications of adoption might be touched upon as well as the checking of documents.

The complaints by magistrates, that their guardians' reports made dull reading and yielded too little information, might in part account for the speed with which the courts did their adoption work. The Hurst Committee observed that the enquiries of the guardian laid too much emphasis on material conditions, and there was a tendency for the far more important factor of the emotional relationship between the child and the adopters to be overlooked.[1] The examination of nearly 300 of these reports during the course of the survey confirmed this and emphasized the magnitude of the courts' task in trying to sift through the mass of detail. All those aspects which could have made for understanding of the particular case seemed to be absent. Moreover welfare authority reports were rarely included with those of the guardian and the number of statutory visits actually paid was not recorded. The courts were therefore not always in a position to judge how well the children's department knew the applicants and child. Had they known (or thought to ask) that sometimes fewer than three visits had been paid (according to the records) they might conceivably have dealt differently with the work.

The Hurst Committee concluded that inadequate reports were

[1] Hurst Committee, p. 20, para. 75.

due to the use of unskilled or unsuitable persons as guardians.[1] But as in the selected area only skilled and experienced child care officers were appointed as guardians, a further remedy seems necessary. The more detailed directives[2] supplementing 'The Particular Duties of Guardians',[3] as well as a closer link between courts and children's departments, would perhaps help.

Finally a particularly intractable problem needs to be mentioned: namely, the court's difficulty in knowing what action to take in cases where it is felt that an adoption order will not promote the child's interests. Once an order has been made, the child, like any other child, could only be brought back to the juvenile court on the grounds that he was in need of care, protection or control. This includes neglect or cruelty. If the case is found proved the court may commit the child to the care of the local authority on a fit person order. There is no provision for removing a child from applicants where adoption has been refused. There are three types of case in which supervision, having once begun, continues until the child's eighteenth birthday. One is when notification of intention to apply for an adoption order has been given but the applicants change their minds and never lodge an application though they keep the child. Another occurs when an application is made but subsequently withdrawn or allowed to lapse. The third type is when an adoption order is refused by the court. In those instances where orders were granted despite the children's departments' reservations, the decision was probably reached by the courts for one of two reasons: either because the circumstances indicated that the child would remain with the applicants whatever the court's decision, and on balance it seemed better to give him the security of status he would otherwise lack; or because it was likely that if the order were not made, the child would be uprooted and this might seriously threaten his sense of security.

In the absence of follow-up studies it is only possible to speculate on the consequences of making orders where the omens are not too favourable. But the writer wondered how far courts in

---

[1] Hurst Committee, p. 20, para. 75.

[2] The Adoption (Juvenile Court) Rules 1965 require that the *guardian ad litem*'s report includes 'such other information, including an assessment of the applicant's personality and, where appropriate, that of the infant, as has a bearing on the mutual suitability of the applicant and the infant and on the ability of the applicant to bring up the infant.'

[3] Adoption (Juvenile Court) Rules, 1959, Second Schedule.

the selected area were aware that where they refused to make an order the children's departments had the duty to continue supervision. These doubts were strengthened by the discovery of several children in respect of whom applications had been refused, who should have been supervised, but were not in fact so protected. Until research sheds light on the consequences of both granting and refusing orders, children's departments and courts might perhaps make more use of this alternative.

8

THE POST-ADOPTION PERIOD

BESIDES describing the events leading up to the adoption, the adoptive parents all commented in more general terms on what their adoption had meant to them. Childlessness and infertility, mixed families of own and adopted children, and the particular qualities of the adoptive relationship were all topics which they willingly discussed. All adopters devoted a large part of the interview to the question of telling the child he was adopted— the one issue that inescapably forces them to recognize their own and their child's special status. The second part of this chapter is concerned with this subject.

The majority of the agency-sponsored adopters were unable to have children of their own or to add to their family. Most therefore, had to face their infertility and this, according to many of those interviewed, was their greatest challenge. Certain adopters made only fleeting reference to their feelings on this and they alluded to the 'second-best' aspects of adoption only indirectly. Adoptive fathers in particular tended to be reticent. One or two suggested that their wife's feelings were paramount, childlessness being principally her loss. But some couples expressed themselves fully and frankly and it was apparent that time had done little to deaden their pain. Many wives, although fully aware that pregnancy was impossible, nevertheless admitted that they could never still their longing for a child of their own—despite their conscious realization of the immense happiness and joy which their adoption had brought.

However, a fifth of the agency-sponsored adopters had 'mixed' families with own and adopted children at the time of the placement, and ten of those families seen had children of their own. Only a few of those with mixed families claimed that the absence of the blood tie was irrelevant. 'I can't help you much on that, he's our own just like the other one, and we never think or feel any differently.' Yet even those adopters who were able to say that their feelings for all their children were identical did not claim that difficulties were absent. For instance, other people were often curious about how they felt towards their various children, and specifically asked about this. Few adopters were untouched by these and many other questions, explicit and implicit, to which all said they were exposed. Neither could relatives and friends be relied on to view adoption in the same light as the adopters. Many reported that their adopted child had been treated differently in some way by other people. Whatever the adopters' own confidence, none ignored the probability that amongst their children there would be more than ordinary cause for rivalry. Indeed this was said to have arisen particularly where older children were concerned.

In effect, most adopters admitted that a mixed family had created certain additional worries, and that they had found their feelings were not, and could not be exactly similar. This difference was claimed to be more than the normal variation of feelings that parents experience towards their different offspring. Adopters had had to learn to face this, although they found it hard to locate the precise difference or to judge how far-reaching the consequences might be. Some believed that neither their adopted nor their own child had an inkling of the different quality of their parents' feelings. However, those who feared that the adopted child would eventually feel differently loved thought that the real problem would be to prevent him from exaggerating or misunderstanding this difference. As one couple said rather sadly, their efforts to be scrupulously fair in all things and at all times could not wholly protect them from fears that their adopted child would occasionally see himself at a disadvantage.

But though most of those with mixed families claimed this had increased their anxiety, it did not follow that they agreed with those societies who consider all applicants with one or more 'own' children ineligible. On the contrary, they all felt that all the children stood to gain, given adopters who could cope, and they felt they had learnt to cope. A mother who already had two boys of her own when she decided to adopt summed up the advantages thus: 'having own children means you've got experience. You've learnt that because they're born to you, you don't automatically love them at once or all the time. They've taught you how different they are, that they'll develop as individuals, and that there's no point in either forcing them, or in expecting too much. Your own children can behave so badly, and hurt you so much, that they'll render you proof against anything. So when your adopted child turns round and says "I hate you", he's *not* meaning "I wish you hadn't ever adopted me". It's less painful to learn from your own children that at times they all believe that their parents are "unfair" and that they're not loved. And just as important as these lessons is the tremendous bond of friendship that has sprung up between our three. It will convince Joanna, if need be, that she belongs and that she's no different. This is going to be as important as anything we, as parents, can prove by our actions.'

Nearly all adopters felt that a family of two children was the ideal size. Only children, particularly only adopted children, were considered to be at a great disadvantage (although this occurred in fifty-eight per cent of agency-sponsored adoptions at the time of placement): just because they were so much wanted they were believed to be more difficult to bring up successfully. In mixed families, there were comments on the relative merits of having an own or adopted child first. Either situation was held to be advantageous to the adopted child. The four couples who had unexpectedly had a child after adopting one were specially grateful to their adopted child, believing their hopes had been fulfilled through him. The popular theory that the care of a child was a remedy for childlessness was well known.

It was frequently maintained that adopted children were often better loved and cared for because they had been wanted so much. Parents who 'bore children regardless, unwanted and unloved' were cited, and several adopters shared the view that 'just because you've given birth to a child, that doesn't automatically make you into a good parent, or prove your fitness'. Whereas most adopters likened their love for their child to that of any good parent a few felt bound to say there was a difference. In their opinion, nothing could quite replace the bond between a child and his natural parents. Therefore they felt their adopted child had a special and permanent need for extra love to compensate him for his loss. These views seemed universal and appeared to be translated into a desire to provide their adopted child with 'only the very best'. Many had indulged in lavish material care and the importance of this was linked with the generally shared view: 'It's no good taking on more children than you can care for really well.' Indeed only one couple out of the whole sample had adopted more than two children, but because of the policies of some agencies there were fewer opportunities for adopting a second or third.

It would be difficult to prove whether adopters' aspirations are higher than those of other parents. But most of those who were seen clearly had considerable ambitions for their child, and these featured prominently in the interviews. Many saw their child's potential as above average. Milestones were claimed to have been passed unexpectedly early, precocity in all sorts of directions seemed to be the rule. Even if unusual promise was not evident in school reports, the child's interests or hobbies were frequently offered as proof of exceptional gifts.

As many adopters said, and as all implied, adoption had not merely altered the child's life: it had transformed their own to an even greater extent. 'When people say our children are lucky, I tell them it's *us* who are the lucky ones. When they came, life began again.' Clearly both those who saw adoption as a simple, natural alternative to ordinary parenthood, and for those more conscious of the special features which mark off the adoptive relationship, adoption was a turning point in their lives.

TELLING

'Society is in process of making parenthood a highly self-conscious, self-regarding affair. In so doing, it is adding heavily to the sense of personal responsibility among parents. Their tasks are much harder and involve more risk of failure where children have to be brought up as individual successes in a supposedly mobile, individualistic society, rather than in a traditional and repetitious society. Bringing up children becomes less a matter of rule of thumb and tradition; more a matter of acquired knowledge, of expert advice; and as the margin of felt responsibility extends, so does the scope for anxiety about one's children.[1] Many of the couples interviewed gave this very impression of self-consciousness in their role as parents. In particular, their failure to reproduce seemed to have intensified their need for success with their children. The fear of failure and the scope for anxiety seemed potentially greater than for ordinary parents. Nowhere was this more apparent than when the subject of telling was under discussion.

Adopters were uneasy, whether or not the child yet understood his status. Those who had so far said nothing wondered when to tackle the subject, and how. Those who had brought themselves to the point of explaining (or had been forced to it by circumstances), were concerned about the repercussions. They all felt especially handicapped by the absence of proven experience. The research worker was repeatedly asked about other adopters' experiences.

In accordance with the recommendations of all the agencies and often the courts, the overriding majority of the school-age children were said to be familiar with the word adoption.[2] However, not only the writer, but the adopters themselves often doubted how much the child really understood. Most of the adopters who had told their children prided themselves on having done so. There seemed to be several reasons for their satisfaction. All accepted that it was their duty to enlighten their child, so by saying something they felt they had made the approved move. Moreover, all were ready with stories of children who had become unloving, rebellious, or even delinquent, through being told suddenly or too late, or by someone other than his parents. The solicitous enquiries of friends and neighbours also served as constant reminders that public opinion favoured telling. But the strongest incentive of all was the adopters' lively fear that others might forestall them. The child's right to this information was

---

[1] R. M. Titmuss *The Family*, p. 8. National Council of Social Service, 1953.
[2] Amongst the forty-six adopted children in agency-sponsored families all but thirteen were five or more at the time of the interview. See Appendix 3, Table viii, for ages of the adopted children in families interviewed.

mentioned less often, though for a small minority of adopters this was their major justification.

For a few, the practical impossibility of getting away with dishonesty seemed to be the main reason. Typically these adopters were forced to 'tell' by such circumstances as the child's need for the 'long version' of the birth certificate which includes the word adoption. Were it not for such situations these adopters saw no case for telling and no merit in being frank; the child could only stand to lose from the disclosure.

Who had done the telling, and when? Fathers played a minor role and few were present when the child had first been told. It was generally the adoptive mothers who had taken the initiative, and it was they who decided when the time was ripe. Outside circumstances had played an important part. Admittedly most children had been introduced to the word adoption and to the 'chosen' concept[1] when bed-time stories were told. Frequently however, this approach had led nowhere as the theme was not developed. One of two later events had galvanized adopters into more effective action: the arrival of another adopted child, or the approach of school.

The eighteen couples who had adopted a second child had found the preparations useful in broaching the subject to their first: 'We're going back to the nursery where you came from, to chose another baby.' Though it was claimed that telling was easier this way, the children did not necessarily appreciate the distinction between being adopted and arriving more convention-ally. Thus one child, on learning that a neighbour was expecting a child asked, 'Is she fetching her from the nursery where I came from?' At the time of the interviews few second adopted children had yet been told, although several had passed the age when the first had been deemed old enough to understand. 'She's less advanced.' 'He's that much more sensitive.' Some adopters seemed to hope that the elder child would relieve them the task of enlightening the younger.

Adoptive mothers felt a child should not be under the double strain of learning that he was adopted and of having to start

---

[1] For example see *What Shall we Tell our Adopted Child?* issued by the Standing Con-ference of Societies Registered for Adoption which discusses the 'specially chosen' concept.

H

school. For this reason, and the conviction that their child was bound to find out once he mixed with other children, many felt they had better take preparatory action beforehand. Several however waited until the very last moment.

Although adopters held that telling ought to be dealt with naturally and informally very few had found this to be possible. Only rarely had a child's comments or questions been used as an opening cue. One child saw a film about the birth of animals and then asked about her own origin. Her adoptive mother said, 'I wanted to lie. I nearly did, but I knew if I didn't tell her the truth then, I never would. She'd never believe me, had I had to go back on what I'd said.' In creating the opportunity and coming to the point the embarrassment and anxiety of many adopters was still apparent long after the event.

About a third of the children seemed to have been told they were chosen 'because you were the sweetest'; or 'the one who smiled', or 'the one we loved best'. This 'chosen' concept, advocated by numerous societies, was rarely linked with a statement about another mother. Some adopters turned their back on this detail. 'We told her, you didn't have a mummy. And we didn't have a little girl. And so we chose you, and you made us so happy.' However many adopters had deliberately rejected the 'chosen' approach. In their view it was not only inaccurate but, more seriously, they felt such stories could mislead the child and perhaps even make him feel inferior. How should he reconcile having been given up with having been chosen, anyway? Adopters who favoured more realism believed it was as important to refer to the 'other' mother (and sometimes also to the father) as to introduce the word adoption. Some children were said to have grasped the essentials well before other parents deemed that a child could possibly be old enough to understand. Thus some five and six-year-olds were said to have understood the exchange of one set of parents for another: yet some eight and nine-year-olds were 'obviously much too young yet'.

There were considerable differences of opinion on how far questions should be induced or encouraged, and on what amount of detail should be given and when. While most declared themselves ready to deal with some questions, the writer's impression was that once adopters had done what they thought was necessary the onus shifted to the child. In discussion little mention was made of any questions children had asked, and there seemed to be a tendency for adopters to associate lack of questions with lack of interest. The writer felt that the amount of help or explanation given to the child by adopters was related to the degree of interest reported in the child. However questions about the natural mother predominated. 'Why didn't my other mother keep me?' 'Didn't she love me?' 'What was she like' 'Where is she now?' Quite different images had been created in the children's minds. Some adopters referred to 'your real mother', or 'your other mother'. Others preferred a more remote frame of reference, 'the lady . . .', 'the person . . .'. The child's illegitimate status was indicated by some, ignored by others. 'Your mummy had no daddy to bring home the pennies. So she had to go out to earn and couldn't look after you, and you came to us.'

Some children were said to have put very searching questions to their adopters about their origins, the rest showed an alleged lack of interest. The results of a recent survey of adult adoptees may be relevant here.[1] The subjects of this study recollected that as children they had been most curious about their origins. They wanted information about their 'real' parents, but it had to come from their adopters. The adopters in their turn awaited their child's questions, and in their absence assumed that nothing need be said. The children had kept from their adopters the turmoil within them, but though they feigned indifference they resented parental attitudes which implied that they were not old enough to understand, or that the details were not their concern. Where information was withheld, or reluctantly given, or accounts conflicted, they had concluded that something significant was being hidden.

In the few families visited where the adopted child was approaching his teens, more adopters reported interest in the subject of adoption. For instance, a twelve-year-old had had several discussions on the wisdom of looking up his natural mother, and in another family where foster children were often received, illegitimacy, fostering, and adoption were freely dis-

[1] A. McWhinnie, ibid.

cussed. Amongst a few of the younger children too, adoption as a subject was sometimes kept alive through the conscious endeavours of the adopters. 'We feel that it's important they should not forget—which might easily happen. Both our children have two anniversaries, their birthday and the day they came to us.' The distinction was drawn between 'always harping about it' (which was considered undesirable), and letting the child feel that it was a subject that could be discussed.

A small number of adopters reported that their child had been upset at being told he was adopted. In three of these cases the disclosure had occurred at school and the adopters felt guilty that their child had been shocked and distressed, although one adoptive mother whose child 'ran home crying his eyes out, so upset' concluded that if this was his reaction she had better leave the subject alone.

Whether teachers should be informed was a moot point. The large majority felt this was important for the child's protection. A few were afraid of discrimination. In small communities however the whole matter was felt to be out of the adopters' hands: 'everyone knows'. As for the children's own part, most had been counselled to say nothing. 'It's something special, a secret just between ourselves.' Rarely did they feel free to say, as one couple did, 'It's up to him to tell whom he likes'. Exceptionally, a child had shared the news freely. 'She's told everyone—she's very proud.'

In only two instances was it quite clear that children were being purposely misled. One of these was dropping hints that she was seeking confirmation of her doubts: 'Mummy, did you go to bed when I was born? Did it hurt?' Her adoptive mother said 'I can't bring myself to do it. Mary isn't old enough (at eight) to know. There's another adopted girl in the village who's bound to be at the root of it.'

Of all the groups of adopters seen, the highest proportion who had told their child he was adopted were in the agency-sponsored categories. Yet it was in just these groups that there sometimes appeared to be less realism and less forthrightness than amongst the other groups. Only a minority of them felt able to deal with this matter confidently. Plenty of explanations were offered for this, and even those who had tackled telling fully and frankly often argued against the stand they had taken. First and foremost, adopters made it clear that they could not bear to shock or hurt their child, or to give him the chance of feeling in any way at a disadvantage. Telling was seen by many as deliberately courting this risk. All text books, as one adopter pointed out, stress the child's paramount need for security. Was she not, therefore, justified in saying nothing while her child was young; surely such telling and creating a sense of security were simply not compatible? Many others seriously doubted their child's ability to understand, and they rejected the advice to 'tell the child early, so that there would never be a time when he had not known'. It was not simply a question of understanding adoption. Telling was seen as essentially linked with giving the facts of life, and for the illegitimate child this meant introducing him to the concept of unmarried motherhood. 'You'd only muddle him how, and tell him things he should know nothing about.' Because of this interrelation, a number of adopters held that it was quite unrealistic to suppose that information could or should be retailed little by little. Hence their reason for prevaricating.

Though numerous adopters stressed their child's inability to understand, they were nevertheless much preoccupied with thoughts about what their child might think of them once he knew. Concern on this score certainly seemed to have reinforced the adopters' reluctance to tell, though few admitted it directly. One adoptive mother who had had to stint and scrape wondered whether her children might think her mean, or that later they might feel that they would have been better off elsewhere. Disciplinary questions were felt by many to present greater problems to adopters than to other parents. There was some anxiety not only as to the child's attitude to punishment, but also occasionally about the reactions of neighbours. The adoptive mother of a disturbed ten-year-old described a situation that several adopters dreaded. She felt the child had set her natural mother on a pedestal, and that she was her rival. Moreover, as the child had made various accusations against her adoptive parents their position in the village was not an easy one.

This fear of not being thought as loving or kind as the natural parents was certainly common, and not restricted to mixed families of own and adopted children. Speculations as to how the child might view them led adopters to wonder how they ought to represent the natural parents to their child. Doubts on this score had also increased the difficulties of telling. Both the amount of information adopters had and their attitudes to what they knew, had determined what they told their child. Though most felt that they knew too little, a few said they were handicapped by knowing too much. For instance, how could a child be told that his mother was married; would he not feel much more rejected than if he had been illegitimate? How should one explain to a child that nothing was known of his father? What should he be told about his natural brothers and sisters? 'We've been able to give him a good home, love, married parents. But we've not been able to give him back his brother and sister.'

Adopters whose child was of local origins felt that the practical repercussions (if not now, then in the future) made their problem specially acute. Questions as to whether it was politic to tell the child his 'real' name or to allow him to see the adoption certificate which gives the place of origin, could not for long be regarded as academic. Several adopters felt this would be the ultimate test. A few suggested hopefully that the child would not be interested. Many more however, showed that they disagreed with the statement: 'though many adopters worry about it, it is rare for a happily adopted child to wish to look up his adoption records, and even more rare for him to try to find his first parents. If they do, it usually means that something has gone wrong in their home and they are searching for a satisfaction that they have not found.'[1] These adopters did not feel that curiosity was a reflection of failure. They anticipated that interest would naturally mount with approaching adulthood. 'I know if it were me, I'd want to find out everything.' Indeed an adoptive father who was himself adopted had followed this very course.

One or two prepared for the event by trying to influence their child against his natural parents. 'I'm not one who believes in telling a child his mother couldn't afford to keep him. I've told him, his mother didn't want him.' Likewise, another had informed

[1] Jane Rowe, *Yours By Choice*, p. 147. Mills and Boon, 1959.

the child: 'your mother didn't want children, but we did.' Only a very small minority felt it necessary to resort to such tactics. More felt that a child should not under any circumstances have the chance to feel that he had been rejected or that he had been the cause of difficulty—matrimonial, financial or any other. They wanted the child to feel that his natural parents had been loving parents whose one concern was the child's happiness, even if this did not exactly coincide with the facts. But this, in turn, raised other doubts in adopters' minds. If their attitude to the natural parents was too sympathetic, might this not have the result of encouraging the child to seek them out even more resolutely! In this and other apparent dilemmas about telling, adopters were uncertain: they had many doubts and some misgivings. They found it difficult to decide with confidence on the 'right course'.

Records and interviews testified to the efforts that had been made by the adoption societies and the local authorities to prepare adopters to deal with telling confidently, realistically and positively. However in view of the difficulties adopters encountered, the conclusion would seem to be that the amount (or the timing) of the help given had been insufficient. Many had not yet come to terms with telling; moreover, the widespread demand for the research workers' reassurance, the incidence of practices which seemed potentially harmful, as where natural parents were being actively discredited, or where illegitimacy was ignored, all suggested that adopters needed yet more support. Too many had failed to appreciate that first and foremost, telling was their problem, not their child's.[1] Without this insight there was little likelihood of resolving their dilemma.

As was pointed out in an earlier chapter, supervision coincided with a time when applicants were not really free to listen because they were identifying with 'ordinary' parents, and because they saw themselves as being on trial. And, all too often, the period of supervision was very brief. Could more have been done to relieve the natural and inevitable anxieties arising out of telling? Apart from the obvious possibilities of intensifying the contact with applicants before and after placement, and perhaps of lengthening

[1] See H. David Kirk *Shared Fate: A Theory of Adoption and Mental Health.* Free Press of Glencoe 1964 for a discussion of the adopter's acceptance and rejection of their special role.

the period of supervision, the suggestion has been made that 'adopters would be visited by the same person who placed the child both during the probationary period and, occasionally, if the adopters were willing, after the adoption order had been made'.[1] Many adopters remembered having been invited to return to their agency should they ever need advice. None had done so, though a few maintained a link by sending donations or photographs. Although there seemed to be an unmistakable hesitation to seek advice, their response to the survey interviews showed that if others took the initiative adopters welcomed the opportunity for discussion.

Numerous American and Canadian agencies have developed the idea of a voluntary post-adoption service, and apparently the response has been very encouraging.[2] Particular interest has been shown in series of group meetings for adopters who want the chance to discuss topics of mutual interest, such as telling, sex education, and illegitimacy. Such gatherings have not only been found of immediate interest and help but have also led some adopters to re-establish contact with their agency. Equally, they have provided the staff who run these groups with ideas for improving their service. It is worth noting that these groups were instigated because caseworkers had become convinced that much of the discussion pertinent to the child's future adjustment had fallen on deaf ears during the period of supervision. Certainly several adopters and officials seemed to feel that some form of voluntary after care service, including group meetings for applicants and for adopters, should be available in this country, too.

[1] Hurst report, p. 13.
[2] See for example, 'After Adoption' Betty Woodward, in *Children*, July-August, 1957.

9

DIRECT AND THIRD PARTY ADOPTIONS

DESCRIPTION

A 'DIRECT' adoption is one where the natural parents have themselves selected their child's prospective adopters. 'Third party' adoptions are those in which natural parents place their child with prospective adopters through the help of an intermediary person who acts as a go-between. Where no distinction is made between these two types of placement they are referred to below as private adoptions.

Subject to certain regulations, parents are free to place their child for adoption with whom they wish, and to enlist the help of a go-between. But 'bodies' as distinct from private individuals are legally disqualified from participating in adoptions unless they are a registered and licensed adoption society.

The incidence of private adoptions in this country is not known, hence regional comparisons cannot be made nor trends established. The Registrar-General's tables differentiate between related and non-related adopters; the latter may be either private or agency-sponsored. In 1954 it was thought that about a quarter of all orders made were in respect of agency sponsored applicants. The Hurst Committee states, '... even allowing for those cases where the child is adopted by a father, mother or relative, there is no doubt that more than a third of the adoption orders made annually are in respect of children placed outside their own families, either direct or by third parties.'[1] In the selected area it was found that the incidence of private adoptions differed markedly from the number that had been expected. They accoun-

[1] Hurst report, p. 12.

ted for only seven per cent of the orders granted during the four year period. Eight were third party adoptions, and fourteen were direct placements, a total of twenty-two of the 295 cases studied.

It seems to be the view of adoption societies and local authorities that adoptions which are not sponsored by an agency are undesirable, and that their incidence should therefore be reduced. The alleged danger is that the child's needs may not be given primary consideration. Indeed, his needs may not be the focus of interest at all: the benefits to the proposed adopters, or the mother's need to relieve herself of the burden of a child she cannot care for, or does not want, may be the major consideration in making the arrangements. The likelihood of an unsuitable placement is said to be all the greater because neither natural parents nor third parties have the skill, or the experience, or the means that are available to adoption agencies in selecting adopters and in matching the child to the home.

Though no comparative studies of the different types of adoptive placement have been made, the Hurst Committee recorded that 'almost all the witnesses we have examined... have stressed the undesirability of third party adoptions'.[1] There was less comment about direct adoptions, though in the selected area they were almost twice as numerous and they were (in the writer's opinion) subject to many of the same limitations. But despite representations that restrictions should be placed on private adoptions, the Hurst Committee felt it would be neither wise nor practicable to prohibit them. Were this done it was feared that *de facto* adoption might grow and even less control or supervision could be exercised. The number of private adoptions investigated in this study was small and hence conclusions about their success or the problems which might arise are somewhat hazardous. In any case it was not the writer's purpose to measure the success or failure of the adoptions that were studied, but to consider the adoption services in relation to the various types of placement.

Before discussing private adoptions further it is useful to give a few details about the children, the adopters and the natural parents involved. The twenty-two children concerned had been

[1] Hurst report, p. 11.

adopted by nineteen couples. Fourteen of the families were visited. Three of the remaining five had left the district, one family could not be traced, and the fifth failed to reply to the letter inviting survey participation and was therefore presumed to have refused.

The children adopted privately did not appear significantly different from those adopted in other ways. All but two were illegitimate and eighteen (eighty-two per cent) were under six-months-old when placed for adoption. Only two were more than a year. A much higher proportion of them (seventy-seven per cent) went directly from their mothers to their adopters than was common with either adoption society or local authority place-ments (twenty-six and thirty-eight per cent respectively); and fifteen of the nineteen adoptive couples knew their child's natural parent(s) personally.

Nine of the nineteen adoptive couples were known to have been turned down at least once by an adoption agency.[1] The adoptive mothers tended to be older than those who received children through an agency, indeed nine of them (forty-one per cent) were forty or more. Only fifteen per cent of agency-sponsored adoptive mothers were as old as this. There also seemed to be a tendency for these adopters to be of a higher social class than any of the other groups. Only one was classified below the registrar-general's social class III (skilled workers) group. Comparisons of proportions are made in Table 15 below, but these must be treated cautiously since the number of private adoptions is small.

So far as the natural mothers were concerned, they tended to be slightly older than those in the other categories. Only one was under twenty and two thirds of them between twenty and twenty-five. The median age of the whole group was twenty-four-point-three. Almost a third were married, divorced, or separated. Over a third (thirty-six per cent) had already had an illegitimate child (and half of these had had two or more) at the time of birth of the child included in the survey. Twelve mothers were in full-time employment, and five were housewives.

[1] Four of these private adopters had previously adopted a child and seven were known to have adopted another after this particular adoption.

TABLE 15

Social class of different categories of adopters

	Registrar-General's social class			
	I and II	III	IV and V	No Information
	%	%	%	%
Private Adopters	41	46	4	9
Local Authority	12	45	39	4
Adoption Society	34	51	7	8
Mothers adopting own	15	49	31	5
Relatives adopting	–	74	22	4

THE LOCAL AUTHORITIES' EFFORTS TO REDUCE THE INCIDENCE OF PRIVATE ADOPTIONS

The children's departments in the study area had pursued a definite policy of trying to reduce the incidence of private adoptions. As ultimate responsibility for a child's placement rests with the natural parents (particularly of course with the mother), they were the chief targets of the local authorities' campaigns advocating the value of agency-sponsored adoptions. But since a third of the private placements had been arranged by third parties, these 'agents' were also included in the plans to reduce the number of private adoptions.

It may well be a mark of the success of the local authorities' policy that agency-sponsored adoptions so greatly outnumbered those privately arranged. However, it was impossible to discover whether natural parents who chose to proceed privately did so deliberately (to retain greater control over selection for example), out of ignorance of the available services, or because they had found it difficult to have their baby accepted by an agency (like some of those who had already had previous illegitimate children).

The main direction of the children's departments' efforts to reduce this type of adoption lay in encouraging better co-ordination between all those agencies that natural parents might contact when planning for their child: general practitioners, health visitors, moral welfare workers, and maternity and hospital staff. At the same time efforts were made to discourage individuals who were known to act as third parties. As one example of these co-ordinating efforts, a children's officer described monthly meetings held with moral welfare workers. Their purpose was to review plans in hand for all unmarried mothers to ensure that they had the help they needed for themselves and for the coming baby.

As the general practitioner is likely to be the first person to whom a mother turns and as he might indeed be the only professional adviser with whom she makes contact, children's officers had actively drawn the attention of all doctors in the area to their services. Doctors were particularly asked to refer any mother who wanted to discuss adoption plans to the children's department as soon as possible. Sometimes this meant that help had been made available sooner, giving more time for the discussion of the alternatives to adoption, for drawing the mothers' attention to the relative advantages of agency-sponsored adoption, and for making plans.

Attention was also paid by the children's departments to obstacles which, it was suspected, might deter a mother from using the available services and thus from placing her child through an agency. For instance, it was feared that some mothers turned down mother and baby home vacancies because admission is, in some cases, conditional on a set period of residence before and after confinement, regardless of the mother's wishes. One children's officer had successfully negotiated admissions where this rule had been relaxed to suit individual needs. Other efforts, aimed at promoting a less rigid approach towards meeting the unmarried mothers' needs, included discussion with local homes and hospital wards that made breast feeding compulsory, again regardless of a mother's wishes and plans for her baby. Closer liaison with medical social workers and ward sisters was aimed at.

Of the eight children in the sample placed by third parties, four had been found homes by doctors, and two by others connected with the medical profession. There was lengthy correspondence with one doctor who had arranged a series of placements. Eventually, he was confronted with chapter and verse evidence of the unhappiness and anxiety that had resulted from his actions. The two survey sample children whose adoptions he had arranged were each placed within the area of his practice. The concern of both the natural and adoptive parents when they discovered this was a factor with which he cannot have reckoned. The two couples each told the writer that earlier on they had not realized the degree to which they would be handicapped by entering into private adoption arrangements. In particular, the question of how much to tell their child filled them with trepidation.

The writer felt that further measures to combat private placements merited consideration. Of the children placed by third parties, only two out of these eight intermediaries had given the local authority the required fourteen days' notice of the proposed placement. Ignorance or evasion of the law may have been responsible. Though the Hurst Committee said, 'we hope that local authorities will take more active steps to ensure that the requirements of the law are widely known. One of the best methods of obtaining publicity is by prosecution . . .'[1] none of the local authorities reviewed had in fact chosen to exercise these powers. Prosecutions could serve as a valuable means of drawing natural parents' and adopters' attention to the risks involved in private placements.

Additionally, homes and hostels for unmarried mothers might consider the appointment of a consultant caseworker to supplement the help given by visiting child care officers and moral welfare workers. This would ensure that many more mothers knew exactly what the statutory and voluntary agencies have to offer, and that they could all count on having the necessary advice and support. Ideally all unmarried mothers, whether admitted to a home or not, should be guaranteed the help of one trained worker able to offer continuity of advice and support right through the period of pregnancy, and for as long afterwards as her situation demands.

The need for publicity, particularly in the form of specialized literature, appears to have been almost wholly neglected. For instance, there was no evidence of books or pamphlets for natural parents or for adopters, setting out clearly and simply the advantages of agency-sponsored adoptions over those privately sponsored. Neither were there publications drawing doctors' attention to the work of the adoption agencies. As innumerable adopters pointed out, local authorities and adoption societies do far too little to make their work known.

[1] Hurst report, p. 13.

THE LOCAL AUTHORITY'S SUPERVISION
OF PRIVATE ADOPTIONS

Where a thitd party proposes to place a child for adoption, he must, by law, give the local authority fourteen days' notice so that the children's department can satisfy itself that the home is suitable. Where natural parents arrange the placement themselves, no official notice of the transfer need be given until the applicants decide to proceed officially with the adoption arrangements. The degree to which local authorities can exert influence on natural parents and on applicants is, of course, more limited where adoption plans have already been agreed by the parties. Six of the eight third party placements were made without the statutory notice having been given, and in two instances in particular, though the local authority was very uneasy about the mother's arrangements, they had insufficient grounds for taking the matter to court.

Locating children placed privately was described as a perennial problem by the child care staff. Two of the adopters seen admitted that they had delayed the official notification of intention to adopt for fear the child might be removed by the 'authorities'. These adopters felt that the children's department and the court would be less likely to oppose their plans if the child had had time to become well established in the applicants' home. The more time the applicants gained, and the longer they had to prove the excellence of their care, the more hopeful they were that their right to the child would be self-evident and therefore established. They clearly hoped possession was nine-tenths of the law.

The interviews and the case records studied showed that nine of the nineteen private adopters had been unsuccessful at least once in applying to adopt through an agency, not necessarily because they were unsuitable. Occasionally the same local authority that undertook statutory supervision had been one of the agencies that had previously rejected the applicants. Though this rejection was not usually associated by them with an individual, but rather with the agency, there were two sample cases where the same child care officer had been involved in both rejection and supervision.

No doubt these factors reinforced the general concern expressed by child care officers in supervising this category of adopters. The staff felt that they had too little scope to prevent such placements and too little hope of influencing either the applicants or the outcome of the application. In several cases the staff were aware that their visits met with hostility, and that they were only tolerated because they were backed by the arm of the law. The realization that their efforts on the child's behalf were hardly regarded as helpful by the adopters made them feel that this was perhaps the least rewarding part of their work. Nevertheless, as Table 11 shows, particular efforts were made to offer as much protection to these children as possible, and it was in respect of this category that the highest average number of supervisory visits were paid.

THE NATURAL MOTHER'S CHOICE OF PRIVATE ADOPTERS

Natural parents were not invited to take part in the survey for reasons given in Chapter 2. Consequently this discussion of their motives for proceeding privately is largely based on supposition. There were however, many clues to be found in the files of the children. And as more than half the private adopters knew their child's natural parents personally, another useful source of information could be tapped.

A mother's readiness to dispense with agency help can be interpreted in three ways: she may be ignorant of the services available, or of their value; or she may see positive advantages, for herself or her child, in remaining self reliant; or she may prefer this course because of negative attitudes to the agencies, or to the idea of asking for help. All three considerations probably help to explain how these twenty-two children came to be placed without recourse to agencies.

Since opposition to private placements is shared by many of the professional people with whom unmarried mothers are likely to make contact, and as public opinion also seems to favour the belief that adoptions are 'best left to the experts', it may be assumed that many of the mothers who placed their child privately knew that agencies existed, and also that private adoptions were viewed with mistrust. Nevertheless, when assessing the use made of the social services, the role played by ignorance should not be underestimated. For example, numerous adopters in all categories complained that they lost time trying to find out about the range of services that exist. Similarly, several private adopters admitted to the writer that they had not appreciated at the outset the degree to which they and their child would be handicapped by the difficulties inherent in private placements. Yet others seemed to have employed the services of a solicitor unnecessarily. It seems more than probable that some natural parents as well were unaware of the services offered by the various agencies. In particular, where natural mothers felt speed was important, or had delayed action and created something of an emergency, ignorance of the services, or difficulty in locating help may well have been relevant to the decision to proceed independently.

There was some evidence, however, that certain mothers took this decision deliberately as being the only means that afforded them some peace of mind. In the matter of choosing their child a family for life these mothers felt that it was essential that they trusted to their own instincts. If they were to delegate responsibility to an agency three sets of strangers might be involved: the agent who enquired into the mother's circumstances (probably a moral welfare worker); the agency that accepted the child (about whose methods the mother would probably know little or nothing) and the adopters (whom the mother would probably not meet and of whom she could not therefore approve personally). This reluctance to trust others to safeguard their child's welfare was well illustrated in the case of the couple who placed their sixth (legitimate) child with friends. They are recorded as saying that they would not have parted with this child to anyone else and were adamant that they would not have anything to do with any adoption agency. The natural and adoptive fathers had served together in the Army. Their wives had known each other at school and at work. Both parties had mutual confidence, and respected each other's integrity and motives. Similarities of background and upbringing meant that matching presented no problems.

The confidence that sprang from personal knowledge of the adopters was likewise illustrated by the fully documented views of a young professional woman who also said how essential it was to her that all the major decisions regarding her illegitimate child had been in her own hands. To give herself time to consider her plans, she initially suggested a temporary fostering arrangement to the couple she located through an advertisement. The transfer took place when mutually convenient. She had been at hand to supervise the child's settling in and had satisfied herself that all went well. Having seen that the family was good and kind, generous and warm-hearted, she could 'rest content' and asked the couple whether they would like to adopt the child. Though, as she said, she had chosen for her child a less affluent or privileged upbringing than her own family might have provided, she was happy to have placed her child with these applicants of her own choice. She had been able to determine just how much the adopters should know about herself and about the child's father, and had taken what steps she thought necessary to ensure that the adopters would later tell the child her reasons for the adoption decision.

Apart from the natural parents' need to feel satisfied about the plans made for their child, there were two further considerations equally relevant to the parents' decision: namely, speed and certainty in completing the adoption plans. These objectives are allegedly more easily secured by private placement than via agency-sponsored adoptions. That speed and certainty had indeed been crucial was borne out by the number of mothers in this category who were working full time; the number who were married; the number who had one or more children to support; and the number who, because they were older than the average in the sample, could probably not fall back so readily on their family for help.

Almost every one of the case files of these twenty-two children showed how important speed had been. For example, there was the married woman who had admitted to her husband at the last moment before his demobilization that she was expecting a child that was not his. His readiness to forgive her was conditional on the child's immediate placement for adoption. This mother was probably aware that several adoption societies (though not all) refuse to place a child for adoption before the age of six weeks; and that her own admission to a home (which was made necessary by her husband's attitude) could well mean a compulsory stay of several weeks. Likewise, this mother may have been swayed by the consideration that agencies, or agency applicants, may reject a baby or return it; a threat which is thought to undermine morale in homes for unmarried mothers.[1] By keeping responsibility for their child's placement in their own hands, natural parents would at least know exactly where they stood.

There was more difficulty in obtaining evidence of other reasons for by-passing the adoption services; but the comments of mothers who had adopted their own illegitimate child were often relevant. Their experiences of the social services, and their attitude to the help offered (discussed in Chapter 10), shed indirect light on this question of private placement. Their accounts suggested that current attitudes towards illegitimacy as well as fear, ignorance and misunderstanding, all had a bearing on the decision to act independently. Though public opinion about unmarried parenthood is perhaps less censorious than formerly, there is no doubt that there is still a great deal of prejudice. Many who had reared their own illegitimate child said that they had encountered criticism and rebuff, which reinforced their own feelings of guilt and inadequacy. Several had either suppressed their need for help or else they had postponed the decision to admit they were pregnant for as long as possible. Indecision may have been one reason why mothers were slow in seeking help, in case they were 'rushed' into a course of action they might regret. Sadness about the adoption decision may have made mothers prevaricate until they believed it was too late to approach an agency.

Some mothers felt that help was made too conditional and their fears on this score may also have explained why agencies were by-passed. These fears were not entirely without substance. Some mother and baby homes, for example, limit admissions to 'first' cases only. Certain of the adoption societies reviewed will only help mothers with their first illegitimate child, and others will not accept third or subsequent illegitimate children. Some, regardless of circumstances, will not offer help with adoption plans where

---

[1] For instance the form natural mothers are asked to complete and sign by one adoption society contains a clause: 'If for any reason, the arrangements for adoption do not materialize, I understand that I can be held responsible for removing the child from the Society's care.'

the child is legitimate. One mother whose child was in the survey sample and who described herself as a prostitute was refused admission to a local authority mother and baby hostel on the grounds that she might have a bad influence on other younger women: partly for this reason she intended to place her child privately with adopters, and would have done so, had not unforeseen circumstances led to the baby's admission to the care of the children's department. The religious sponsorship of moral welfare workers may also be a factor limiting a mother's readiness to seek help.

There were several aspects of private adoption which seemed disadvantageous to the natural parents. Knowledge of their child's whereabouts appeared to be a terrible and exacting price to pay for the advantage of private placement, notwithstanding that it was probably this very consideration that made some mothers decide that they must select the adopters themselves. The temptation to see their child even after adoption, to find out how he was getting on, and whether his care was adequate, had proved too much for several of those in the survey sample. According to the adopters, this knowledge of the child's address caused some mothers acute anguish, and robbed them of their peace of mind. One mother called monthly, sometimes more often, at the adopters' home. Another regularly sought information through a go-between. A third was said to be known to her child as the adopters' 'friend': on certain days, at a certain cafe, the parties meet 'as though by chance'.

Natural mothers who acted independently had a more restricted choice of adoptive homes for they were normally limited to a range of people known either to themselves or to their agent. A less easily substantiated drawback for mothers was that the adopters they had chosen lacked an agency's approval. True, they knew that the court's ultimate approval was required and had been given. But they were without the assurance that some form of critical selection had taken place. Perhaps most worrying of all, these natural parents had foregone the opportunity of discussing their adoption plans with an independent experienced adviser. The consequences of this could be far reaching, as illustrated by the account of one of the adoptive couples interviewed. The natural mother of the child they adopted had been 'let down' by the father. When the mother proposed adoption to the applicants, they persuaded her to enter into agreement: on discharge from the maternity home, she would accompany them to their solicitor. There she would agree that the applicants should, in due course, adopt her baby, that she would not change her mind, and that she would not interfere. The adopters said that their 'most helpful' solicitor had drawn up this agreement and that it had been duly signed. They did not say whether it was made clear to the mother that the document was not legal and therefore not binding. The *guardian ad litem* had known nothing of this arrangement.

THE ADOPTERS WHO PROCEEDED PRIVATELY

The visits paid to the fourteen families who adopted privately underlined the difficulty of making any generalization about them. There were certain features however which did create a pattern. Amongst these was the fact that the two parties were usually known to one another and did not live far apart. As a result, a complete break between them did not occur when the child was placed. This seemed to be accepted as inevitable, though not desirable, by the adopters. Hence there was at least the possibility that the child's loyalties might be divided. In the light of this the adopters felt that their task of explaining his adoptive status to the child was particularly difficult. Only half had been rejected by adoption agencies, but all seemed conscious of official disapproval. Consequently, they hardly felt able to make full use of the supervisory period, and regarded the children's departments with suspicion.

One case history serves to illustrate several of the above features.

Young Mrs Jones needed help and advice about her divorce, which was imminent. She knew that the complicated structure of the family living opposite was due to the fact that both Mr and Mrs O'Casey had been previously married: there were children of three different unions living under the one roof.

Following Mrs Jones' divorce she became more friendly with Mr and Mrs O'Casey, especially when Mrs Jones found that she was expecting an illegitimate child. A few weeks before her baby was due, Mrs Jones informed the health visitor that she would be placing the child with Mr and Mrs O'Casey for adoption. At that time, after paying her rent, Mrs Jones' total income for herself and her young children was very low: but in a year or so, when her youngest had reached school age, she would be able to go out to work full-time. Meanwhile, she was doing her best on her National Assistance allowance. She told the child care officer that she could not face the long postponent of earnings which would be inevitable if she kept the coming baby, 'it was not fair to the other children'. Hence her decision to place this child with Mr and Mrs O'Casey, who declared themselves wholly agreeable. Mrs Jones was emphatic that she would not part with the child to any adoption agencies. She *had* to know where and to whom her child was going. Mr and Mrs O'Casey had not previously thought of adoption, but in the circumstances (according to Mrs Jones) they said they very much wanted to complete their family, admittedly already rather large, by becoming this child's parents.

Mrs Jones asked the child care officer for no help other than for confirmation that her plans for her baby were legal. The case file entry records a joint interview with Mrs Jones and Mrs O'Casey, aimed at bringing home to them the difficulties that might arise if the natural mother and the adopters still lived so close together. Mrs O'Casey realized, as a result of this discussion, that she would have to think again about the feasibility of 'bringing the child up as though he were her own and best that it should know no different'. She was able to appreciate that if she didn't tell the child at an early age, neighbours might, but said that if, as was hoped, they were rehoused, 'this would make everything easy'. The child care officer was told at this visit that Mrs Jones only knew the putative father as a casual acquaintance, he was not aware of her pregnancy and she did not wish him to know.

As it happened, Mrs O'Casey acted as midwife to Mrs Jones. When the child care officer paid her first visit to the prospective adopters five weeks after the baby's birth, Mrs O'Casey was not only caring for the child, but for the mother, too. Mrs Jones was still perfectly agreeable to the proposed adoption. At this visit, the child care officer learnt that some time in the future, Mrs Jones was going to marry one of Mrs O'Casey's sons by her previous marriage. If the adoption order was made, this would mean that the child's brother by adoption would also be her natural mother's husband and her uncle by adoption.

On this visit the child care officer again tried to make clear to the adoptive applicants and to the natural mother, who were seen together, some of the complications which would ensue were the adoption order made; particularly the child's difficulties of divided loyalties. In an effort to convey the realities of the situation the child care officer asked the natural mother to imagine her feelings were she to see her child maybe chastised by the adopters while she herself stood by. Mrs Jones retorted that even if the court did not grant an order to the adopters, her child would remain in the care of Mr and Mrs O'Casey as long as they were prepared to offer the child a home. Once again, she confirmed her right to place the child with applicants of her own choosing. She was warned that, in view of the circumstances, the court might well feel that it could not make the order, or that an interim order only would be granted in the first instance, in view of the continued close contact between herself and the child and the adoptive applicants.

Only one further home visit is recorded prior to the application to the court, which took place when the child was just a year old. The *guardian ad litem* reported that the child had a very loving home and that the applicants wished to adopt from the best of motives. But the guardian recommended to the court that, because of the unusual nature of the relationship between the applicants and the child's natural mother, particularly because of the proposed marriage between the natural mother and Mrs O'Casey's son by a previous marriage, 'which would make the infant's natural mother also her half-sister-in-law, it is respectfully recommended that an adoption order should not be made at this stage, as such an order might well lead to a very real confusion in this child's loyalties as she grows up'.

The guardian informed the court that the applicants intended to keep the child as a foster child if the order was not made. The court decided in favour of the applicants, and the order was granted despite the children's department representations.

When the research worker called on the adopters five years after the making of the order, she met not only Mr and Mrs O'Casey and the child, but also Mrs Jones' second husband, Roy. He was a frequent visitor to his parental home. The adopters had arranged for him to be present, knowing that he was anxious to discuss his domestic situation, particularly his parents' adoption of his wife's illegitimate child. It emerged that his marriage proposal to Mrs Jones (as she then was) had been conditional: Mrs Jones had had to choose between him and the child; if she wanted marriage, then the child (whose father Roy had known well) had to go for adoption. Mrs Jones had countered this, saying that she would agree to part with her baby for adoption, provided it was placed with Roy's parents as she had no relatives of her own. In spite of Roy's immediate and clear realization of the drawbacks of this counter-proposal, and despite his initial opposition to it, Mrs Jones was adamant that her baby should not go to strangers. Roy felt, and said repeatedly to the research worker, that he felt that if only the baby had gone to strangers his wife would have got over it. But 'she insisted and so I agreed, and my mum and stepfather agreed, and it was done.' 'We never speak of the adoption. But I've seen her tears. I'd hoped it would get easier. I don't believe it ever will. If we'd have some of our own, it would help, but so far we've not been lucky. Of course, she knows, as I know, it's the best way. But it's something you never get over, I realize that now, and so does she.'

Mr and Mrs O'Casey were under no delusion about the cost of a mother's parting with her child, though they never referred to it openly. 'She calls sometimes three or four times in the week. It's only natural, it's her *right* after all, isn't it?' Several times during the survey interview, Mrs O'Casey referred to Mrs Jones as the child's 'mum', though her relationship to the child during the interview provided no other clue that the girl was not one of Mrs O'Casey's own. 'That was the most terrible year I've ever lived through, waiting, just waiting, as to whether they'd give us the baby. We were on the rack, and they put the screws on us. We knew they were against us, they told us so. They tried to talk us out of it at first. But they soon saw it was no use. The health visitor came and was against us too. We've not had any more to do with her after that. She just wouldn't see.'

'There's this question of telling, and that's why Roy wanted to be here when you came. He feels that because *he* forced the issue, he's got to tell the child. He feels guilty about it, so that's why he thinks it's his job. The court advised us to tell her right from the start. But we just don't agree. In fact, I think it's rubbish to tell her before she's old enough to understand everything; not just the facts of life and all that, but how it all was. Until she's got that far, it's no use. I know lots of the people round here know, but just because of that you can't force things into her head that she can't figure out. Of course, we shall tell her everything in the end, we've promised her mum we would, it was one of the first things. Her mum has always made us promise one thing, not only that we'd tell but that we'd make it quite clear that she wasn't one of *those* women. The welfare also told us to tell, but they have no idea what a job it is in this sort of case. Just now, she thinks her mum's her auntie, like the other children. We're glad to leave it at that. As we have been rehoused we feel we can wait a bit. Of course, if she asked it would be different. None of our other children talk about it, and we don't think the youngest know. So that's how things stand, and that's the way we feel we ought to leave it for the time being.'

This case history is clearly not typical. It has been included, however, because it demonstrates some of the disadvantages of private adoption which have been discussed. Other cases did not show these so dramatically or comprehensively.

It might be suggested that adopters who act privately either see no reason to do otherwise because of personal knowledge of the natural mother, or chose this course because they have been unsuccessful in receiving a child from an agency, because they did not meet the eligibility criteria; were thought to be unsuitable, or were still well down the queue. For this latter category who had failed to get a child from an agency the decision to proceed privately may be seen as some measure of their determination and ingenuity. That they tended to be older and of a higher social class than most of the other adopters may also be relevant in this respect.

10

JOINT ADOPTIONS BY MOTHER AND STEP-FATHER

GENERAL CONSIDERATIONS

THE Legitimacy Acts[1] provide that an illegitimate child may in certain circumstances be legitimated on the marriage of his father and mother. But if a mother marries a man who is not the father of her child and wishes him to share her parental rights, then the couple must jointly apply to adopt the child. The Registrar-General's reviews shows that of all the orders granted in England and Wales in the decade 1950-1960, approximately one third were for children adopted by their mother and her husband.[2] The incidence of adoptions by mothers and husbands in the selected area followed closely the trends indicated by the Registrar-General's figures: in the four year period 1955-1958, 102 of the 295 children adopted (thirty-five per cent) fell into this category. Sixty-one per cent of these adoptions were arranged subsequent to the mothers' first marriage. Of the remaining thirty-nine per cent, eighty-three per cent of the adoptive mothers had been divorced and seventeen per cent widowed.

In this category the implications and objectives of adoption differ from the popular concept: as several of the adopters remarked, 'we wanted to change the child's name'. The recognized aim in such cases is to regularize the child's position in the family so that, as far as possible, his status and his rights shall be indistinguishable from those of the children born of the marriage. It might be argued that a study of this category of adoptions falls outside the scope of this enquiry: but there were several important

[1] The Legitimacy Acts 1926 and 1959 and The Legitimation (Re-Registration of Births) Act 1957.
[2] Registrar-General's Annual Statistical Reviews.

reasons for including them. Locally, as well as nationally, this type of adoption is numerically important. Secondly, because of the step-father relationship, these families might be expected to present strengths and weaknesses which would repay special study. Thirdly, as the child care officers said, and as the records confirmed, little is known about the implications of adoption for the different members of these families. Finally, as a result of the legal changes introduced by the Adoption Act 1958,[1] the adopters of this category are no longer required to give their local authority three month's notice of their intentions to adopt: thus, there is now even less opportunity of discovering the needs of this section of the adoptive population.

When selecting the families in this category to be interviewed, all adoptions following a mother's second or subsequent marriage were excluded, as many of these families contained children of three unions. It was felt that the significance of the adoption factor would be obscured by the complex family structure; therefore, the selection was made only from adoptions following a mother's first marriage.

Because of the numbers of adopters in this category who declined the invitation to take part, the aim of securing twenty interviews was modified: only sixteen couples were seen. The following extract from a letter to the children's officer throws some light on the refusal rate: 'Both my husband and I have given much thought to the question of taking part, but I have a particular reason for not wanting to do so. My husband has proved himself more considerate than I ever thought possible. We do not discuss the past and have built up a very happy present and, I hope, future. I feel it would not be fair to him to risk his unhappiness or embarrassment in bringing up past events, and I hope sincerely you will understand.'

All who participated emphasized how greatly they welcomed this opportunity of talking over their experiences. At their own request two couples who were in difficulty over their child's adoption were referred back to their children's officer. In seven instances the writer paid a second home visit in order to discuss the adoption further with the mother alone.

[1] Adoption Act, 1958, Section 3.

Of all the adoptive couples seen, these were the ones who had perhaps had to make the most subtle and complex adjustment of any. They had realized that theirs had not become an 'ordinary' family simply by virtue of the making of the order: adoption had, indeed, solved some problems but it had created others.

MARRIAGE

Their reaction to unmarried parenthood, and their speculations about the future had resulted in months, if not years, of conflict for several of the mothers in this category, before they had felt able to commit themselves to marriage and to its apparently automatic sequel, adoption. Uncertainty at this stage had been a feature in the lives of all the mothers, even though such privileges of marriage as status, security and companionship had indeed held particular attractions not only for them, but also for their father-less child.

Certain mothers had initially rejected the idea of marriage as being contrary to their child's interests. They feared that the child-step-parent relationship might assume its proverbial form. 'When Jack was small of course, all would have gone smoothly. But once he understood his father wasn't his real father, what then? It was up to me to make sure they'd both be happy. We were courting for five years.' In the child's interests, a prolonged courtship had been considered essential by almost all the adoptive mothers seen. The few relatively speedy marriage decisions were almost always commented on regretfully during the survey, so far as the child's adjustment had been concerned.

Outside circumstances had helped several mothers to agree finally to marriage. 'My dad was father and mother to me. His death was partly what decided me, because I didn't feel I could manage Vera without him.' 'My father and brother were killed in a crash. My mother had always been against my keeping Jean, so quite suddenly I made up my mind and said "Yes".' Considerations about the child's best interests featured prominently in these mothers' accounts. No comparable information was obtained by the writer about the adoptive fathers' attitudes to prospective marriage.

Concern about the step-father's acceptance of their child was but one point on which mothers had needed repeated reassurances. Understandably, it had been at least equally vital for them to know that they themselves were acceptable despite having had, and kept, their illegitimate child. Naturally, this was one of many points on which most mothers were reticent. But one mother remarked: 'My husband often says he respects me more for having stuck by Diane through thick and thin, than had I let her go, as my relatives advised. It's been a special bond between him and me, and such a comfort.'

Both during courtship (and beyond in some instances) the fiancés (or husbands) had had to compete against powerful forces. In private, several mothers admitted how tenaciously the past held them back from giving themselves fully to the future. 'Not till I heard that Hank was repatriated did I learn to stop longing for him.' Another said, 'Of course, marriage has made me very happy. But I yearned for the terrific intensity of feeling that Poppy's father called out in me. I knew what a fool I was, and what his true feelings were for me, and how he behaved when I said I thought I might be pregnant. But in spite of all that I couldn't put him out of my mind, especially not with Poppy there constantly reminding me of him.'

Although forty-five per cent of the adoptive mothers in this category were less than thirty years old at the time of their marriage, several admitted to difficulty in making the change. Almost all had been in full time employment prior to marriage. 'Having responsibility, an organizing job, and financial independence for eight years, I found marriage quite hard going at first.' This mother had achieved independence in the teeth of adversity. Marriage to a man fourteen years her senior had meant 'retirement' to a routine secluded life which was in complete contrast to all that had gone before. No less than one in five of the adoptive mothers in this category married a man at least ten years older than themselves. Possibly this, too, had reinforced doubts on the advisability of marriage and adoption.

ADOPTION

Of the sixteen couples who described their experiences, only one had not seen adoption as an inevitable and natural corollary of marriage. The sharing of legal responsibility for the child had been regarded as 'right and proper', to be arranged as soon as possible. All the mothers said, or implied, that they had wanted to share their rights in recognition and acknowledgment of their husband's role. The latter may have been equally eager to proceed, adoption may have been a symbol of their acceptance of wife and child. The common sense aspects of these adoptions, the search for status, respectability and completeness, had each heightened the sense of urgency. That the interviewed couples were representative in this particular respect of those not seen is borne out by the statistics. Thirty-six per cent of applicants in this category adopted when they had been married for less than one year; and no less than seventy-two per cent of the orders were in respect of couples married for less than four years. In the four other types of adoptions combined, only seven cases (four per cent) involved couples married for as short a period as this.

The statistics indicate two obvious motives for speed in finalizing these adoptions. One quarter of the couples had other step-children, and it was in the interests of the child to be adopted so that his position would be regularized. And forty-two per cent of the couples had had a baby in the interval between applying to adopt and being granted the order. Several of those interviewed confirmed that it was the advent of a child of the marriage that had made them feel they should hurry on with adoption plans. Regret that circumstances necessitated adoption and reluctance to reopen the past were additional incentives to 'getting the adoption out of the way'.

Only a minority commented positively (or indeed in any way) on the adoption process itself. The most favourable remark about supervision was 'that it was good to know that people (i.e. the children's department) cared enough to come and call to see how you were getting on'. Generally, adoption was regarded as a mere formality; the legal ratification of an already existing situation. The value of supervision and guardian's visits was minimized. 'It was just to check that we understood that in future we'd share the child legally.' They had had no doubt that the order would be granted. The records confirmed the accounts of those interviewed, that there were fewer discussions than might have been expected on the deeper implications of adoption, such as about sharing the child, or the step-father's attitude towards a non-related child, or the particular difficulties of telling in this type of adoption. Not until much later had some of these adopters realized that their circumstances were unique and that therefore there was a case for supervisory discussions.

THE POST-ADOPTION PERIOD

Though these couples only referred to their child's adoption briefly, the achievement of their goal, namely the child's integration in the family, was no less vital to them than for any of the other adopters seen. Interests and concern centred, of course, on the relationship between step-father, child and mother. These adopters seemed particularly sensitive about this, no matter how well they appeared to have adjusted to marriage and adoption. However, taking part in the survey probably sharpened their awareness of, and preoccupation with, this question of family relationships. These couples drew attention more openly to their special situation as adopters than did any of those in the other categories.

Most of the adoptive fathers acknowledged that they did not feel the same to their wife's child as their own children. All but one of the couples seen had 'mixed' families. Generally, the fathers felt that it was they, rather than the adopted child, who stood to lose from this special relationship. All but one of the stepfathers doubted how far as yet, the child saw himself at a disadvantage. They, on the other hand, regarded their own position as a difficult and tenuous one vis-à-vis the child. 'I can't cuddle her; she won't let me, even when she was small she wouldn't. She'll only come to me when her mother's out.' Several expressed regrets of this kind. References to disciplining the child made it clear that this was another area in which difficulties had frequently been encountered. Similarly, those mothers who had spent long periods rearing their child unaided said that they had found it hard to learn to share him. Inevitably, the difficulties here were common to all three parties the older the child the more difficult it was to modify the pattern of relationships. The mothers (and some of the adoptive fathers too), had had fears that stepfathers could not as easily understand the child, that they might expect too much, or that their methods were foreign to the child. Excessive leniency and spoiling on the adoptive father's part were commonly reported. This made some mothers more anxious, whilst for others it strengthened the bond.

The arrival of a child of the marriage was nearly always claimed by both parents to have reassured them about the adopted child's place within the family. At the same time, their comments showed that it also reinforced certain anxieties. For example, this event seemed to have sharpened concern about the adopted child's reactions to 'telling'; in particular its impact upon his relationship to his adoptive father and his siblings. Even where this hurdle had been overcome, or where circumstances obviated the need for explanations (because the child was of an age to understand when the order was made), there was still anxiety amongst step-fathers: what was their standing in the child's eyes?

The mothers' feelings were also important. The few interviews conducted with them privately were of particular interest. As one admitted, 'Often I find myself having to take sides and it worries me. It's like a tight rope act. I feel so grateful to my husband. Yet I'm having to defend my child against him sometimes, which might *seem* natural enough, but in the circumstances it's different.' When the going was hard, one or two mothers admitted that they could not help but think back occasionally to the advice that had apparently been commonly given at the time of the child's birth. 'Don't stand in his way: what have you got to offer him, you *owe* it to him to give him up.' As they said, they had no regrets. But their path was not smooth.

Feelings of guilt about having had an illegitimate child had obviously not been wholly resolved amongst this group of mothers. Some were affected to quite a marked degree. As one said, 'every time people remark how much she's like me, I wonder how much they know and whether they're getting at me?' Another said, 'I can't stop myself from blushing every time there's mention of illegitimacy, broken homes and unmarried mothers, and so on. It seems to come up so often.'

The relationship between mothers and daughters was said to

K

afford particular scope for anxiety. An adoptive father felt sure their task in enlightening the child would have been easier had it been a son and not a daughter to whom the adoption had to be explained. 'A son would make more allowances.' One mother said, 'Anne is now a teenager: I ought to be talking to her about whom to go out with and what time she's to be in by. But then I say to myself, who am *I* to lay down the law to her, what does she think of me, what *can* she think?' Rather helplessly and despondently the mother of a girl who had made her need for more control very obvious said, 'The one thing above all else that I dread is that she'll also have an illegitimate child. I'd rather anything than that. I shan't feel safe till she's married.'

These problems were harder to deal with because the mothers felt unable to confide fully in their husbands. There also seemed to be a sense of isolation from their relatives. In numerous instances, the mothers' parents no longer played their former helpful role. 'Mary was practically brought up by my parents. Without their help, I shouldn't have been able to keep her. She still spends most weekends and holidays with them. So in a way she's their Mary and mine, and the other children are ours, my husband's and mine.' Gratitude for past help perpetuated what several mothers recognized as anomalous and trouble provoking situations, whereby they still felt under an obligation to share their child. Though some saw that their relatives were undermining the cohesion of their family, they felt that the remedy was beyond them. In one or two instances, the relationship between a mother and her parents-in-law had been permanently blighted by the explanations about the child's existence when marriage had been first proposed.

In this category in particular, adopters said it was the chance to talk over the problems of telling that had led them to take part in the survey. In their view they were up against greater difficulties than other adopters. Eight of the sixteen couples interviewed said their child was in ignorance of his true relationship to his adoptive father. The remaining eight 'knew' although only one of them had had to be deliberately enlightened: the rest had been old enough to understand when the order was made. Indeed sixty per cent of all the children in this group were already over five when adopted. This is significantly older than in all other categories of adoption.

The adopters who had as yet said nothing were only too conscious of having gone against the advice they had been given. They were harassed, in case others forestalled them. Even so, not all acknowledged that their child was yet old enough to understand, although all were by now of school age. What had deterred them? The impression was gained that these couples were less willing or able to discuss the problem of telling with each other, and husband and wife more frequently held different views on the question.

The child's ability to understand and to be discreet had to be taken into consideration; also the fact that the mother would be implicated morally in the explanation if she had been unmarried. Her dilemma was obvious. All said they felt compelled to tell their child something of the truth even though they feared the consequences of telling, as much for themselves as for their child. They realized only too clearly that, having once mentioned the fact of adoption, sooner or later the child would be bound to ask questions about his 'real' father. The mother's problem was to decide what to divulge, and how and when to proceed. The belief that their child would be more sympathetic and tactful, and that he might be content not to press for information once he was older, helped endorse their views that delay was best. The adoptive fathers also appeared to favour postponement. In fact, most of them thought that the middle or late teens would be the best time, and in this, differed from their wives who generally suggested that telling should be done sooner, before the child reached secondary school age.

The adoptive father's wish to protect his wife was one obvious explanation why delay was advocated. But equally important and representative were the following views expressed privately by one mother: 'Whatever *my* views on telling, there are also my husband's. I know he's hamstrung by stories about cruel stepfathers. Frankly, he's afraid of losing her love once she finds out. He could not bear anything to come between himself and her. He keeps thinking of children who turn round and say, "you're nothing to do with me". He loves her and spoils her, and she couldn't wish for a better father. And yet he's afraid.' The fear of losing the child's love was obviously a potent deterrent to telling. It highlighted the difficulties that these adopters felt they were up against. All thought that the task was infinitely easier where neither adopter was related.

Understandably, it had been difficult for adopters to know how best to broach the subject of the natural father. Almost invariably the mother felt that the task was hers. Particular courage was needed and usually it was not until they felt they were 'cornered' that they brought themselves to the point. One mother described such an event. 'Two months ago, when the two of us were alone, my (thirteen year-old) daughter suddenly broke down. She was ten when she went to court, but we'd never discussed anything. Eventually she admitted that she wanted to know about her father. I'd been wanting to tell her, but I'd never been able to get started. I was glad she made me. I expect she'll want to ask more about him later. I'd much rather she came out with her thoughts. Just then, my husband came in. I don't know how he guessed what we'd been talking about, because he and I rarely discussed it. But then there were hugs all round.' Two mothers described how their child too, had forced them to face up to the issue. Two others, on the contrary, had forestalled their child's questions by making it clear that the subject was closed. Both felt guilty and uneasy about it.

The husbands and wives seen all clearly needed help and reassurance. But, as many pointed out, they felt that the persons best equipped to help were similarly placed adopters who had had actual experience of their particular problems. This category was particularly avid for news of the experience of other couples, and they regarded the idea of occasional group meetings for adopters (on a purely voluntary basis) with particular interest.

THE CHILDREN'S DEPARTMENT'S VIEW OF ADOPTIONS BY MOTHER AND HUSBAND

In the chapter on supervision issues of general importance to all types of adoption were discussed. Here the aim is to concentrate briefly on the supervision problems particularly relevant to this category of applicants. The child care officers' difficulties in helping parents to make constructive use of the supervisory service were highlighted in descriptions of their efforts on behalf of mothers and step-fathers. In effect, the staff doubted how far, even if applicants wanted help or advice, it was possible to offer it at that stage and within the available time. The majority of the staff felt that effective supervision of this category was a goal rarely if ever achieved, and most of them disliked this part of their work.

In many cases the period of supervision followed closely on marriage. Fifty-one per cent of these couples had been married less than a year when the order was granted and supervision had typically started from three to six months earlier. Hence the new pattern of relationship between mother, stepfather and child was still only in a formative stage. Thus, as child care officers pointed out, supervision could have run its course before the implications of adoption had had time even to emerge; before the mother fully realized what sharing her child meant; before the step-father knew how he felt about taking on another man's child, and how he felt towards that child; and before the child's reactions had had time to crystallize. These children were, it will be remembered, significantly older than the rest. Only thirteen per cent were less than one year old at their parents' marriage and forty-five per cent were already three or more. Naturally the older children were harder to integrate. At a time when most of these families were undergoing a period of major upheaval and readjustment it was hardly feasible to explore the deeper implications of the adoption.

A further obstacle to getting to know the applicants well and to helping them turn their thoughts from immediate considerations to future aspects of adoptions, was the fact that a high proportion of mothers in this category (forty-two per cent) were known to be pregnant during the supervisory period. The advent of a child of the marriage reinforced the applicants' wish to dispose of the adoption as speedily as possible and, according to the child care officers, made the adopters resent intrusion all the more. Their sense of urgency and their wish to keep the matter private often frustrated efforts to be helpful. But perhaps the biggest obstacle for child care officers was the adopters' fundamental attitude to adoption: they were said to see it as a mere formality. Those who had been unmarried mothers might have formed unfavourable attitudes to the social services and all of them had needed to be independent in the past. Moreover, as many of them were seeking status via adoption, it was unlikely that they would be receptive to the idea that adoption in itself would not put everything right. Factors like these help to explain an unwillingness to confide in child care officers. The inherent difficulties in these adopters' situations, as well as the child care officers' difficulty in establishing contact, hardly suggested that arrangements for supervision were adequate. The difficulty of being able to see both parents on their own as well as together was also said to jeopardize the whole aim of supervision. It should be noted that in this category the recorded number of home visits gave reason for concern, as two thirds of the families had received only two visits, or sometimes less. That statutory supervision has now disappeared altogether in these cases must surely give some cause for disquiet.

One possible explanation for this apparently limited contact with the applicants was the fact that visits were not always recorded. Another was the child care officers' feeling of inevitability about these applications: according to them, orders were invariably granted. Their uncertainty about their mission was another likely explanation, for this was even more apparent here than with other types of applicants. The child care officers also queried how far their intrusion was warranted or worthwhile when the pattern of relationship was barely formed. They were unsure about the validity of their advice on the all important question of telling because advice depended on an intimate knowledge of the applicants and their circumstances, and because in any case they were unsure what help and advice was best. Lastly, they felt it was particularly difficult to foresee what might arise in the future, and did not wish to precipitate applicants into discussion of problems which might never arise.

To illustrate some of the points discussed in this chapter, a shortened version of one of the research interviews is given. The account was particularly valuable as it was possible to interview the mother on her own, and she expressed herself more freely than perhaps she would have done in her husband's presence. It is based upon post-visit notes; it was not taped nor were notes taken at the time. As she thought that hers wasn't a 'proper' adoption, Mrs Bee said first that there didn't seem to be much point in my coming to see her. But on hearing that her sort of adoption was indeed of special interest, she quickly agreed. Her son, Billy, was nearly eight at the time, and she was just eighteen when he was born.

We all used to shut up when my father came home from work. He didn't ever seem to care about anything, so long as he had his peace. I was relieved that my mum agreed to tell him that I'd got into trouble. I knew she was suspicious. I used to feel so rotten, and she used to watch me, but didn't say anything. In the end, she asked me straight out, one evening when the rest had gone to bed. I hadn't been able to tell anyone up to that time. I must have been nearly in my fifth month, and my ankles swelled up so that I couldn't do my job. I *had* to go to the doctor then to get a certificate. He told me I'd have to stop off work for two weeks. Of course, all the family had to know all about it then, and I couldn't have kept it quiet much longer, anyway.

I had to have another two weeks off work after that, found I'd lost my job, and couldn't get another. So my mum went out to work, and I looked after the family instead. I never talked to my father about it. The others were told by my mother to leave me alone. I wasn't too bad. I didn't go out much, except for the shopping.

My mother made me go back to the doctor. He told me that our hospital didn't take unmarried mothers for confinement, and that I'd have to be booked in at the next nearest, fourteen miles away. I was too ashamed to question this. In any case, I couldn't bear to go to him. He wasn't the sort you could talk to. Going over for fortnightly checks to the hospital where I'd been booked meant a journey of an hour and a half each way, and a change of bus and a wait. My mum was working full time them. She only came with me the first time. When the lady almoner saw us, she and my mother decided that adoption was best. I just cried. Then, later, my mother wrote to the almoner, as she could see that it grieved me just to consider adoption. They all said it was best for my sake, as well as for the baby's. They thought I was being stubborn. So I just wouldn't talk it over with them, as they were all against me. But I knew from the start I wouldn't let my baby go.

When I had another five weeks to go, and was having a check up, the doctor said I had to be admitted then and there. I wasn't even allowed home to get my things. It was very awkward; in the end my father brought them the next day. The sister told me I had to be *Mrs* Kay. They didn't know that I wasn't having anything more to do with the baby's father and that he didn't *know* I was expecting. In any case, I heard later that he'd been repatriated. Not that the hospital asked. It was the loneliest time I'd ever had. I'd not been in hospital before, or away from home for that matter. Being *Mrs* meant that I had to keep explaining why I hadn't any visitors. It would have been easier not to have had to pretend. Being in so long meant that there were always new patients, and more explanations. Because of the journey and her work, my mother could hardly ever come. I looked forward to the baby a lot. At the same time, I often felt very miserable and ashamed. Sometimes I didn't know what I thought about it, or what I wanted to happen.

They didn't give me any anaesthetic. I was alone in the labour ward for what seemed ages. I knew what the sister thought of me. It was so awful that I swore I'd never go through it again. I was very frightened and I didn't think I could stand it. Though I wanted the baby, when I was in labour the only thing I could think of was that this was what the baby's father had done to me; and he didn't even know what I was going through! In a way I was proud. And I was glad, too, that the baby would be all mine. But it hurt a lot and I was never so alone. I'd rather have been at home.

The almoner only came to see me once after I had Billy. She never asked me anything about how I would manage. She just said: 'I hear you've decided to keep him', and when I said 'yes', that was it. She offered me some clothes, but I'd knitted everything.

I was the only one in the ward without a husband, and the only one never to have a man visitor. My mother came when she could, but she had to leave the children in the waiting room and that meant she couldn't stay long. And with the journey, and the weather, it wasn't worth it, though she did what she could. Some of the other mothers in the ward were nice to me. I think visiting times were worst.

It was marvellous to get home. My mother went out to work again, and I looked after Billy and the family. I was very proud of him and pleased to take him out. I'd been told to go to the National Assistance Board, but even so, I found I couldn't really manage to pay my way, and got myself an evening job from 6-10 p.m. That was fine, except that I lost my milk and Billy didn't do well on the bottle at first. When he wouldn't stop crying, my dad used to shout about wanting his peace. He'd made it plain what he felt about my keeping the baby, though after a bit I think he began to see it my way. But we didn't talk about it much, once he knew my mind was still made up.

There were quite a few rows. Then, when Billy was about a year, there was a real show-down. So I moved out to my sister, though she hadn't much room either. But by then she'd had her first baby, and I must say, it made her a lot nicer about mine. She and her husband couldn't have been more helpful. I went out to work full-time then, and I was able to pay for our keep properly. I couldn't get my old job back again, but my pay wasn't too bad, and it was much better than being on assistance.

My sister had been the only one to whom I could talk about keeping Billy. It helped a lot to know that she backed me up. When the almoner said that with adoption I would never know to whom my baby had been given, it had made me absolutely sure I'd never part with him. While I was with my sister, I'll admit that I sometimes felt I *had* been selfish. Her baby had a father. And sometimes I was scared that I should have to let him go because I might not manage on my own. But even then

I never considered that I could part from him, or that it could have been really right, and my sister knew how I felt.

When Billy was nearly two, my mother was suddenly rushed to hospital. She asked me to go back then, and to look after everyone at home. My dad was pleased that I stepped in, especially as it turned out that my mother was away many months. They all loved Billy, and he was no trouble.

It was then that I started meeting my future husband Robert. We'd been at school together, and then he'd just finished National Service. The second time he took me out I said, 'I suppose you'll have to know, if you don't know already.' Of course he had heard about Billy and that made me feel a lot better, because he took me out knowing Billy and I belonged together.

I was against getting married, because of Billy. I'd always thought that, for his sake, he'd be better without a stepfather. Later though, I changed my mind. What I felt was that Robert never once questioned Billy's place. And it would mean that I could give Billy a proper home and a proper start. I felt I could then make up for what he was missing. Billy and Robert got on fine. Of course, Robert had got to know him well before we got married. And Billy was small, and there was no trouble about him calling Robert 'daddy'.

We'd planned to get the adoption through right away after our wedding so as to get Billy's name changed as soon as we could. When I told my mother that our wedding was all fixed up, that Robert would get a job with a cottage, and that we'd adopt Billy, she was pretty quiet about it at first. You could see she'd still got her eye on Billy. She'd always taken to him, and she wanted him herself. That was what all our rows had been about before. She couldn't help wanting him, seeing how much she'd done for him and for me, and I felt bad about it in a way. It was because of her that I'd been able to keep him, after all. But in the end she saw it my way, and when it came to the wedding, she was as pleased as I that Robert and Billy got on so well. The adoption went through in a few months; there wasn't any difficulty.

It was over discipline and punishment that I realized just

what adoption meant. After I'd had Billy so long to myself, done everything for him, and had such a job to stop others from interfering, it wasn't easy to stand by and see Robert take over. He was strict. Often I felt, as I still do now, that his ways aren't mine. When Mary was on the way, I got pretty worried, wondering how Robert would feel then towards Billy. In a way, Mary helped because I saw that Robert was strict with her, too. And so he is with the babies. But I still think Robert is too strict, and sometimes I know that Billy gets too big a share of the blame. I'm certain that Robert *tries* to be the same to them all, it's what we've always said must be done. But I don't think that a man *can* feel the same to another man's child. He just doesn't understand Billy as well as he understands the others.

Don't misunderstand me. They do get on well. But Billy won't tell his dad much, and then Robert gets angry. I feel the difficulty is mainly on Robert's side. Somehow, he makes Billy shut up like a clam. I've told Robert that probably Billy does sense that his dad doesn't feel as close to him, but Robert won't have it that there's anything in it. It's not something you can argue about. Just occasionally, though, Robert has made me feel that he does know there's a difference in the way he feels towards Billy, compared to how he feels to the other children.

Usually we get by all right. Sometimes I feel I have to defend Billy against his father, and then again, I think of all Robert has done for Billy and me; and then I don't know which way to jump. Sometimes it helps to talk things over, and sometimes I feel it's the worst thing we could do. If Billy weren't such a quiet, shy sort of chap, it would be much easier. But he can't, or he won't, stand up for himself. When he had nightmares about starting school, he wouldn't say anything at first. I had to drag everything out of him. He seemed to think it wasn't all right to be frightened. When his dad is around, he's even more shut up in himself. Robert is sorry about that, but then again he gets fed up with him, and that's just no good. It drives Billy away even more, and Robert just washes his hands of him. I think that grieves Robert as much as it does Billy.

There's one thing that Robert and I just don't see eye to eye about, and that's the business of telling Billy that he's been adopted. We're agreed that we're not going to tell him yet. But only recently, my sister said, '*Isn't* Billy *like* Robert?' and with so many people knowing, and Billy getting sharper, he's bound to wonder what it's all about. I couldn't bear him being told by anyone else but me. As a matter of fact, though Robert doesn't know it, I've been along to tell his teacher, just in case there's any trouble at school. Robert is sure that the day that Billy knows, he'll stop taking any notice of him. Robert thinks he'll *lose,* the day Billy knows, and so he's quite set that Billy shouldn't know for as long as possible. I don't agree with that. I'd like to know what other people in our position think? I don't think that Billy really would change, it's only that Robert is afraid he might.

Billy hasn't started asking any questions about where babies come from and all that, but then he's only seven. It's no use putting ideas in his head, and goodness knows where it would get to, if we did tell him. Not that in a place like this most people don't know anyway. I've made up my mind that it's not for my sake that I'm putting off telling him. It's partly for Billy, because when he knows he might feel different from the other children. And also because of Robert: this is what he wants and thinks best, and so I can't really interfere. But if in another year or two Billy hasn't asked, I shall do something. And if he does ask, I've told Robert that I've got to tell him. I wouldn't lie to him, it wouldn't be fair. But what I'm afraid of is that he might be told by someone else, or even that he knows something now already. I don't know what's right really.

So you see, it's not been all that straightforward, as one might think. But adopting was of course right. We've got by, and the children couldn't stick up better for each other. Billy and Mary are devoted and the two of them are like a mum and dad to the babies. It's that that really makes me glow. And even when we do strike a bad patch, I think of Robert's promise to me, and all that we've gained, and that's what counts. We've come through and we've a good home.

If I had my time again, or had to help someone else, the

thing I'd say first of all is, go and find someone to talk to on whom you can count, someone who's not in the family. I didn't want to talk to our doctor. That was my own fault I suppose. I didn't know anyone else, and apart from not knowing where to look, I was too busy minding my own business. No one told me about Mother and Baby Homes. I had only my relations to talk to about my plans for the baby, and I knew well enough what *they* thought I ought to do. Though if it hadn't been for my mother and for my sister, I might not have been able to see things through at all.

It seems to me that it's only if you're prepared to give your baby away that anyone is ready to help you. If you don't feel that way, and if you're not being helped by the baby's father, you're there, on your own. The worst is that you're not sure if you're doing the right thing, and that is something you do need to have help with, at the beginning especially, when you're making plans and when you're finding out what's happening between you and the father. When you're so low, and ashamed, and you don't feel you can ever go out, it would count for a lot to have someone just to talk to, and someone who doesn't take sides, either. Even now, sometimes, I feel I'd like to talk to someone else in the same position as I am. I don't think that anyone realizes that when you've been an unmarried mother, even if you do get married later, things can never be the same. It's just something you can never really put right. Anyway, I know that that's what it's like for me. Of course, I don't know what it will be like for Billy, or how he'll feel later. And for Robert and me, how we feel to the children can't ever be quite the same: Billy will always be special, one way or the other.

Unlike the case quoted in the previous chapter, this is fairly typical and serves the general purpose of illustration well. Several other mothers expressed similar feelings and sentiments, although their situations were slightly different.

11

ADOPTION BY RELATIVES
(OTHER THAN BY NATURAL PARENTS)

THERE were twenty-seven children in the total sample who had been adopted by uncles, aunts, or grandparents, and sixteen of these related adopters were interviewed. It was apparent that the transfer of a child from one branch of his family to another, and the consequent change in formal relationships, marked these adoptions off from the others. The table below shows the original relationship of applicants to child, as well as the reason given for the adoption.

TABLE 16
Reasons for adoption given by related adopters

Reason for Adoption	Adopters' Relationship to child		
	Grand-parents	Uncles or Aunts	Total
Adoption of child of unmarried mother	8	4	12
Adoption of legitimate child on mother's death	–	3	3
Adoption of child whose parents were separated or divorced	3	4	7
Adoption of legitimate child whose parents had enough children already	1	3	4
Adoption of legitimate child in his financial interest	–	1	1

Many different situations prompted these adopters to adopt the child: 'It was my sister's dying wish that I should bring up her child as though she were my own.' 'My brother and his wife never made a go of it. Their children went from pillar to post. When they separated we were glad to give at least the youngest a decent start.' 'We thought we couldn't have children. When my sister had her fifth, her eldest was only seven. With all those mouths to feed on just a labourer's wage they were more than glad we took the baby off them.' 'My widowed sister was desperate her four children should know nothing of the illegitimate child she was expecting. I was illegitimate myself and brought up in a Home. No relative of mine is going through that if I have anything to do with it.'

In spite of a variety of motives, differences in the children's ages and in the ages of their adopters, this group had one factor in common: the family tie. All confirmed their happiness in having been able to help one of their own kith and kin. Even though some adopters were not favourably disposed to their child's natural parents, this attitude was never carried over to the child himself. The child's membership of the family was obviously valued, as borne out by innumerable references to likeness in looks, temperament and disposition. An elderly adoptive father described his niece as having been an ailing, puny baby. 'They didn't think we'd pull her through. But every night of those first weeks, I warmed her and comforted her on my chest.' As well as the obvious satisfaction they had all derived from the care of their relatives' child, many of these adopters were conscious of having earned the approval of other members of their family.

The satisfactory and satisfying aspects of these adoptions were obvious. The blood tie evidently strengthened the bonds between adopters and child; but there were also signs that the well-being of some of these children was less assured than it ought to have been. Welfare authority and *guardian ad litem* reports, as well as the adopters' own accounts, showed that these adoptions were particularly liable to create a complicated pattern of family relationships from which difficulties could arise. Even at the outset a few couples had doubts about offering adoption for this reason. Moreover, the experiences of some of the children prior to placement, and their age at this time (although twenty were under six months at placement, the remaining seven were all more than two), made certain adopters feel they were at a disadvantage compared with 'ordinary' adopters. Lastly, the security and privacy of some of these related adopters seemed more threatened by the natural parents than in any other type of adoption, except possibly that of private adoption.

Only eight of the sixteen couples seen said they had been fully convinced that it was in the child's interest that they should adopt him. Thus one sprightly young grandmother said, 'When my daughter finally saw that the baby's father hadn't the slightest interest in her or the baby, she was only too glad to accept our offer. She couldn't part with him to strangers, she couldn't keep him herself, and she wanted him to stay in the family, so we were all delighted.' Likewise, the adoptive parents of each of the three children whose mothers had died knew themselves to be the best placed members of the family to offer a substitute home. These children had all spent varying periods with other relatives before finally moving to the adopters.

The other eight couples lacked this certainty of purpose. Anxiety about their own suitability had proved a definite handicap. 'Look at us, we shall be in our late seventies before the boy is through his teens. That won't be much fun for him or for us.' Another grandmother described how, 'I'd prayed that nothing like this should happen to any of our daughters. Yet it did. I was so shocked, I lost my faith. When our eldest broke the news that she was expecting, my husband had just answered Billy Graham's "Come Forward" appeals. I was sure my daughter ought to give the baby up right away, but my husband overruled me. It was up to us, he said, to give the child a Christian upbringing. He gave up his job, his house, his promotion chances, pension rights, friends, everything to avoid the scandal. I tried to warn my daughter what it would be like when he was ours, and no longer hers. I don't think she'll ever get over it. I know how she grieves.' A third couple said, 'At seventeen, our daughter threatened us that unless we consented to her marriage, she'd have a baby and force our hand. We gave in. A year later her husband cleared off. She took up with an old school friend, but his terms were either that the baby went, or his offer of marriage wouldn't stand. So we had the child, as my daughter's husband knew we would. What ought we to have done?'

It was not only grandparents who were unsure of their suitability and the wisdom of their decision. 'My sister and her husband were evicted, and they were going to split up. We'd housed them all at one time or another, and then they asked us to adopt Harry. But though they've gone on separating now and then, they're still married, yet Harry is ours. We've had Mabel and Anne, too, as foster children. But once we realized that the parents weren't really parting, we sent the girls back.'

One in four of the children in this group was at least two years old when they went to the adopters. The latter attributed lasting difficulties to the fact that their adoptive child had not been with them during the early formative years, and also to the experience he had had prior to placement. 'Madeleine came to us in a pitiful state, thin, nervous and shy. She'd nursed her mother nearly to the end and she'd seen too much.' Another of the girls whose mother had died had had more than a dozen changes of home prior to adoption. Children adopted because of the break up of their parents' marriage were likewise claimed to have suffered badly: 'John had been left on his own many an evening, and he came to us terrified. It took us months to sort him out.'

The circumstances which had initially prompted the adoption largely determined the scope for difficulties when it came to telling the child he was adopted. The motherless children, for instance, were all of an age to understand what had happened and to consent to their adoption. Circumstances had enabled four other couples to deal with telling in a straightforward manner, and there was no question of secrecy. However, eight of the children seen had not yet been taken into their adopters' confidence. These adoptive parents were all worried and in serious difficulties. Because the children had been placed as babies, telling had to be undertaken deliberately. Not only had the adopters to face up to the usual problem that disclosure of adoption would inevitably require explanations of the 'facts of life' and of illegitimacy, but as they pointed out, the overriding difficulty was having to admit to 'immorality' or to 'irregular behaviour' within the family. Because of this, they felt telling was much harder for them and for the child than for other adoptive families. As one adopter asked, was any task more delicate or difficult than that of confronting a child with his rejection by a member of his own family, when he still remained within that same family? Three children of those seen were yet to learn that their natural parents were alive, married and living together not far away. Four others would have to be told that their supposed sister or aunt was, in fact, their real mother. These adopters felt trapped and unable to find the right way out of the predicament.

Though these couples were with good reason afraid that others might forestall them, their inclination was to wait until the child could understand 'properly' when he would 'see his adoption in the best light' and 'had learnt how to be discreet'. They argued that by saying nothing as yet the natural parents would be protected, the child saved from confusion and divided loyalties, and their own path smoothed. Apart from their own preference for delay, one or two said that they had to comply with the natural parents' wishes. Thus the couple who adopted their great-niece had been sworn to secrecy. 'Mary's mother, Gwenda, and her husband, come quite often. She hasn't told a single one of the other relations, so *our* telling Mary could make things terribly awkward for her mother. What's more, we believe that Gwenda's husband is Mary's real father, though we've never been told. But when we do tell Mary, isn't she bound to ask, "and who's my father?" Then what do we say when Mary finds out they've got a home and everything?' These adopters were childless and obviously devoted to their charge. Secrecy in accordance with the natural mother's wishes appeared to have been a condition whereby they had secured the child.

Adopters in this category were of the 'opinion that they had more to lose when there were 'real' parents and 'real' siblings at hand. 'We can't face telling her yet: her mother has the child of her first marriage and the three of her second with her. What would Anne think, how could we explain why she wasn't wanted, which was because her parents split up over her birth? It could make her very bitter. The trouble is, everyone round here knows, the divorce got into the papers.' One or two couples faced the future philosophically. Even if the availability of 'real' parents finally tempted the child away they would have had the joy of rearing him. One or two sought to forestall eventualities. 'I point out to James how well off he is here.' 'When I tell David I shall also say his mother didn't want him.'

Nearly half of these adopters felt that for their adopted child's sake as well as their own, it was best to maintain their distance from the natural parents. In several instances a barrier had been erected which the adopters saw as an inevitable, if regrettable, outcome of the adoption. 'I know the price my daughter is paying, never interfering, never showing her feelings. We rarely see each other or write. It's best, for all our sakes.' Several remarked pointedly that their child did not like, did not trust, or had never taken to his natural parents. Or else that the child 'took no interest', or 'never bothered'. Thus, besides changing the relationship between adopters and child, adoption had sometimes also led to a definite shift in the pattern of relationships in the wider family.

Indeed the impact of adoption on family unity had given concern to both the local authorities and the courts. No less than seven of the twenty-seven case files studied showed that the children's departments had either opposed the granting of the order, or that the guardian's report had included reservations on the advisability of making the order. Extracts from two files illustrate the range of considerations taken into account. In one case the Judge, in granting an interim order, told the mother that she must not return to her home—the home of the applicants and the child. At the resumed hearing a year later, the mother admitted that she had not in fact broken contact with her parents or her child. Periodically, she lived with them or visited, '. . . but she says definitely she does not treat the child differently from her younger sisters,' and '. . . she was trying to carry out the Judge's suggestion to allow the child to be the entire responsibility of the applicants and not to interfere.' In another case the guardian 'was not entirely satisfied that indirect pressure had not been exerted on the respondents (the natural parents) by the applicants. The respondents appear to feel under an obligation to the applicants to allow them to adopt, as the applicants had done so much for the child and for themselves (the respondents). The applicants made no secret of their eagerness to adopt the child and the male applicant says that if he loses his daughter (by marriage) then at least he will gain the child. The respondents said they offered to take the child to live with them some time ago, but that the applicants refused this offer.' Apart from the applicants' age and the crowded living conditions, the guardian further commented, 'None of the parties to this adoption anticipate a break between them, and this may well involve the family in the conflicts which are liable to arise when grandparents adopt a grandchild.'

Even at the stage when they were still only applicants, many of the adopters were either already in the midst of difficulties, or else could foresee complications due to their relationship to the child. Only exceptionally however did the accounts of those seen include references to the help given by the children's department during supervision. The impression they gave was that they preferred independence. They saw the adoption of a member of their own family as essentially a private matter.

One particular case study helps to illustrate a number of the points discussed in this chapter. This again was not taped but constructed from notes made immediately after the interview. Any information that could help to identify the family has been withheld.

It isn't until a member of your *own* family has an illegitimate child, that you realize just how you feel. As my sister kept the whole affair secret until quite late on in her pregnancy the shock was all the greater. I think my mother felt worst. And my father just couldn't believe that it had happened to one of *his* daughters. My husband and I couldn't believe it either. Nothing of the sort had ever happened in either of our families. And it was so unlike my sister, anyway.

It was we who took my sister to a solicitor. She just didn't seem capable of making plans. And my mother couldn't face anything. The solicitor had no suggestions to make, though he mentioned affiliation orders, maternity homes and the names of adoption societies. My sister wouldn't hear of court action, and was unsure about adoption. In the end she did agree to apply to a home for unmarried mothers. But when she learnt that to get in she must obey their rule to stay for several weeks before and after the baby's birth, she just refused. My parents were only too willing to pay private nursing home fees—whatever the cost. They were so afraid of gossip, and time was running out. We were agreed that as it was a family affair we should see everything through ourselves. Only our doctor had to know.

My husband and I decided that I should take up my job

again, so that we could support my sister and house her for as long as she wanted to stay and had plans of her own. She seemed quite pleased, but in some way I found that I couldn't really talk to her any more. I couldn't get through to her. We had never before been so remote from each other, and it grieved me. And she didn't seem to care.

Because my own pregnancy made me so unwell, and there was no place in a day nursery, my hopes of helping financially fell through. But we could still offer her room and board for as long as she liked. We wrote to her regularly, by then she had gone away, but we rarely had a reply.

To our amazement, my sister turned down our offer of accommodation for herself, but arrived without warning straight from the nursing home. She had discharged herself early. She just said she wanted to leave Fanny with us, and seemed very cool and casual about it. We didn't discuss plans, except that she was returning to her lodgings and to her job right away.

In effect, I found myself with twins. For my own baby was born just five days before my sister's. My husband and I decided to regard Fanny as a ward in our trust. It was a strange feeling. Though I knew I had her only temporarily I felt that it was up to me to make amends to her for what had happened; for my parents' sake, my sister's and of course for hers. I felt I could do it best by treating both of them exactly the same. Both were equally helpless after all.

So I taught myself to be equal to them. You'd think that when they both start together that shouldn't have been too difficult. I was given every chance after all. And yet it wasn't easy. I hadn't enough milk to feed both, but they shared what there was, and made up with a bottle. I realized I was always going straight to my own baby's cot first, so I made myself take turns. Little things like that helped. As the weeks passed, I sometimes used to believe I really was succeeding, until my husband's example of really true and utter fairness made me realize that, in my heart of hearts, I still had a long way to go.

What always spoilt it was not knowing what my sister really wanted for Fanny. Had I been certain I should have had real conviction. Perhaps the difficulty was that I was trying too hard. And at the time I didn't realize that one could love equally, and yet differently. It seemed a contradiction, whereas now I see that it need not be.

When the 'twins' were about five months old I reached a sort of crisis. I wasn't well at the time; as a matter of fact I was afraid that I might be pregnant again. I wasn't sure that I could cope. I knew that, at first, I had taken Fanny for my parents' sake, because of the shame of it all, because she was related, and for love of my sister. But gradually, as I lost my trust in my sister during those months because of her attitude, I realized I had to re-examine my motives. Until then we two in particular had always stuck closely together. When she had had the baby she changed. It's never been the same between us since.

My religion has always been a tremendous inspiration. Because of my belief I came to realize gradually that the stigma of illegitimacy was not really so important; it depended how you looked at it. I wanted to take Fanny for the love of God. That was so obviously the only right way of seeing it. I was beginning to get irritated with my parents, who were still mainly worried about shame and disgrace. At that time my husband and I felt 'in it' alone, because my parents' feelings became rather irrelevant. Until I'd got my own feelings sorted out again, we were rather apart from them, but later we were closer than ever. Perhaps my parents are still too ready to think of the injuries to Fanny and the disgrace my sister has brought on the whole family. They are of a different generation after all. For myself, I realized that disgrace has very little to do with Fanny, and I hope that shame never will be any concern of hers.

We had become bitter about my sister, I will admit. I, in particular, thought that her indifference had been a cover for her misery. But we realized our compassion was pretty well wasted. The casual way in which she mentioned adoption was probably the parting blow. Until then, she had always given us to understand that later on she was going to take Fanny over herself. At least, that's what we had assumed. We knew that she wouldn't let her go to any adoption agency, and we had never suggested that *we* should adopt her, because we were sure that she would certainly want her own baby, even if at the time she wasn't taking much interest.

Of course we wanted to discuss adoption fully, but she refused to say anything really, except that as far as she was concerned, she didn't want her, and that we needn't worry, she wouldn't change her mind. We had strong suspicions that she was going out with a man who was quite probably Fanny's father. We met them together one day, and the way he picked Fanny up and looked at her gave us the idea.

We saw my sister very rarely. She refused to tell us anything more and we felt it was not fair to press her, even though we felt that we had a right to information as Fanny's future parents. Had I not seen this change in our relationship myself, had it not been me and my own sister, I should have said it was impossible that we should have become so estranged. But you don't understand until it happens to you, what the break up of your family, or of some members of it, can mean. We had always looked alike, and been alike. Now I hardly understood her. And what's more, I despised her, and despised myself for that.

When my sister suggested adoption again, she had waited the month that my husband suggested she should allow herself so as to think things over really carefully. She said she was still perfectly ready to give her up to us for good. We decided we had to get advice. But the moral welfare worker's first comment, that it looked as though my sister had abandoned her baby, made us feel so furious that we felt more strongly than before that we wanted to keep all this to ourselves as our own family affair. When she told us that we had no choice but to go and see the children's officer, we thought that it was outrageous that officials should need to know our private business. Actually, in spite of everyting, quite a number of people on the estate did seem to know though none ever actually said anything. You were never sure who knew what, or what they were thinking. For Fanny's sake, we were in a hurry now to get the position settled; she had become so much one of the family. My sister's confirmation of her plans that we should adopt

Fanny suddenly released tremendous new feelings of love and concern in me; I got very possessive of her. I don't think it was quite the same for my husband, perhaps because from the start he had always simply given her everything he'd got, regardless of the future.

In fact, the children's department could not have been more helpful. Everything from the legal angle was covered by our solicitor and the court clerk. The child care officer who visited was tactful and pleasant, and she obviously wanted to be helpful. Nevertheless, I always had the feeling that it was 'us against them'. I just felt that I could not admit even to the sheer physical effort that was involved and which sometimes proved almost too much. I could not admit that I still occasionally doubted whether I was really loving the 'twins' equally, or that I wasn't always absolutely sure what I really felt about taking my sister's child. Neither did I find it possible to discuss whether we were doing right, and whether we'd be able to see it through right to the end. Fanny would have to know the whole truth one day. Would she feel we had done right by adopting her? If we hadn't been ready to have her would her own mother have stayed by her?

The child care officer was a court representative and a council employee, after all. Were I to admit completely frankly how I felt, it might be decided that I was unstable, or too emotional or over inclined to worry and 'not able to take it'. So we only talked about everyday practical affairs—what the 'twins' had been up to, and the other children's reactions and ailments. In any case, I knew that really major problems only my husband and I could sort out between us. It was we who had to come to terms with them. So there was every reason for me to seal my lips. My husband wasn't usually there when these visits were paid, but we agreed about what was said and not said.

What made us anxious was that we were never sure how far the Council could stop us from adopting Fanny. We feared that adoptions by relatives were specially frowned on, but we didn't dare to ask. Had we not resented interference so much I suppose we would have felt better about it. We didn't realize then that all adopters have to go through the same mill, and that even relations have to accept supervision. Nor did we realize that most applications are granted anyway.

Another point which worried us, and made me guilty, was that our eldest was suddenly going through a phase of really acute jealousy. I found I had to be constantly watchful, or else the 'twins' were in for a pretty bad time. Endless patience and special loving were needed, and eventually everyone was happy again. I never really gave any of the children enough of my time, I'm afraid.

I kept going over my feelings towards Fanny, particularly when I'd had a bad day. The strain of having two fat, growing babies both at the same stage and both so demanding left me pretty drained, even though they were so absolutely adorable and easy, really. Sometimes I was leaning over backwards in trying to be too fair. Mostly I forgot about it and it was much easier. They were so alike yet so different. Sometimes it grieved me to be making comparisons: usually it was a delight. Physically they absolutely flourished. It was just in my own mind that I had fears and doubts.

But one day my doubts as to whether I could really feel towards Fanny in the way I had set out to feel suddenly vanished. I'd been out shopping. My mother, who is nearly blind, had dusted Fanny's bottom with some athlete's foot powder by mistake. As I opened the door her agonised yells greeted me. I saw at once what had happened. As I tore the clothes off her and plunged her in the bath I rounded on my mother. I accused her of the most frightful things, and spoke to her in a way I'd never dreamt of doing before. As I came to my senses, I realized that at any rate there need be no further worries *now*, whether I could develop real feelings for Fanny. They were there all right.

The day of the hearing filled us with anxiety. Not that there was any need to worry about my sister, she had made her attitude to Fanny's adoption absolutely clear. Neither my husband nor I believe, though, that she would ever have let her go outside the family, even though she seemed so casual about it all. She was quite detached, or so it seemed to us. She didn't see much of us and of course didn't come to court. What we were far more worried about was what would happen if the order wasn't made. By then we had had the 'twins' for a year and it was unthinkable that Fanny shouldn't become legally ours, as she was ours already in fact if not in law.

After all that, the hearing was exceedingly brief. To us it seemed fatuous that the Judge should ask if we weren't over-worked or taking on too much. By then the worst time was over, we'd fought all our biggest battles. After all, we shouldn't have applied had we not been sure we wanted her. Both of us felt at a distinct disadvantage standing there before the Judge almost as though we'd done something wrong. We were enormously relieved when it was all over. Had we known how quickly the order would be made we wouldn't have worried so much perhaps.

We're glad to talk over the adoption with you, because from the start it has given us a great deal of food for thought. With friends and relatives, relatives especially, discussion can only go so far; in fact, for Fanny's sake, as well as the whole family's, we prefer not to talk it over with other people. Of course quite a few do know she's adopted, though not, we hope, where she comes from. But between ourselves, we very often discuss our own feelings, and what hers may be later on.

When it doesn't matter, for instance on holiday with people one is never likely to see again, we let the two pass as 'twins', which is easy. So that they wouldn't have too much explaining to do at school we've also let them start as 'twins', and it's at the head teacher's discretion to tell anyone else who needs to know. Quite a lot of the children in their class know. As you saw, I introduced her to you, saying, 'This is our adopted daughter'. She and all our children have got used to hearing that occasionally, as we feel it is a good thing. But we don't overdo it. At the moment we feel it probably doesn't mean anything to her; or at least, we're pretty sure it doesn't worry her, or she'd ask otherwise. We, on the other hand, have worried a great deal about this whole problem of telling. My husband was strengthened in his belief to wait until Fanny is older, when he heard a talk which said, in so many words, let them live it down. But he says that as it chiefly concerns my side of the family I should take the decision.

Both of us want Fanny to know everything. It's only fair that she should. But we are afraid that other people might get in first, and what's more that they might tell her in an unkind or even malicious way. We feel that it won't be until she's in her late teens that she will really understand and we would prefer her not to know until then, because it would be impossible to tell her just so much and not the whole story. If it weren't for the other people on this estate we could well afford to wait. But as it is we feel forced to tell her something now, and maybe it will even mean that we have to deceive her.

We have always believed that a good relationship between parents and children is based on trust. But however we explain things to her, we're afraid she may suffer and feel different even if she's got no cause. It must make her feel different and that, above all else, is what we want to avoid.

Quite apart from that, there's the rift in our family, and we have talked that over time and time again. I don't think I can ever bring back my feelings for my sister, they seem to be shattered. I just don't understand how she could have given her child up like that; nor how she could have married straight away afterwards. And as you know, we are still in the dark about Fanny's father, but have our suspicions. We feel her irresponsibility is proved again, and that she has again put her own interests first regarding her present plans. She promised that she would move right out of the district. But she hasn't kept to it. On the contrary, she and her husband live near enough for us to fear all the time that we might run into them any time. As it is, it very rarely happens. Fanny now knows her as 'auntie', as do the other children of course, but as she sees her so seldom she barely recognizes her. I will say that for my sister, she does keep away, as she said she would. And she rarely calls on my mother either.

What worries us is how Fanny will feel towards her when she knows who she really is. I am ashamed of my feelings to my sister and should feel I had failed Fanny, if ever she realized how I felt. Nor shall we ever let Fanny know that her mother did not want her. But what are we to say if Fanny asks why she didn't keep her? We don't know ourselves. It's so terribly difficult to know what to do for the best. Either she's got to know or we've got to live a lie.

Stangely enough neither of the 'twins' have asked why Fanny alone is our adopted child. Only our eldest did that, and we explained how for a number of reasons mothers sometimes could not keep their babies. They know something about illegitimacy, but none know who Fanny's mother is and we don't propose that they shall know before Fanny herself does. Perhaps it will sort itself out later. But it's a problem we've talked over repeatedly and we never seem to get any further. And yet it's the most important aspect of adopting.

From the beginning we've told Fanny she once had another mother. Perhaps it hasn't occurred to her to question this. We're satisfied that she understands this much. Even before she began school we started on the facts of life, in explaining to her that she wasn't actually born to us, though we were her mother and father by adoption. We've always encouraged our children to feel they can ask any questions. But principles are easier than practice when it comes to explaining irregularities in your own family, and when the feelings of people you love are at stake.

At least we've had no worries about health, or behaviour, or school. Even now people stop me in the street to exclaim about the 'twins', and it is always Fanny who gets most attention. There's no doubt about her good looks, and she's so adorable. It is nice that all our children get on so well together almost always. They're ideal companions and adore each other and they play for hours. It's fun to watch them, they're never bored. Perhaps it's because of that that they're in such demand by the other children; they always think of something new. They practically live out of doors and they're happy all day long. At night there isn't a sound out of any of them.

What I've realized, what we've both of us realized, is that our love for the 'twins' is the same and yet it's different. I can explain it best perhaps, by saying that I love the one because I see as in a mirror all my husband's characteristics, his gait, his mannerisms, everything is so like him and therefore so special. And Fanny I love because she's also my own flesh and blood, she looks very like me; but mainly I think it is because she constantly reveals to me my husband's goodness. I had always loved him deeply. But the way he was prepared to accept Fanny and to help me through those first difficult months made me see him in a different light. Sometimes you don't fully realize even your own husband's depth and strength until you've gone through a new experience together. There was in fact a moment when I felt I couldn't cope. But my husband was like a rock. Come what may, we would stand by Fanny. He has always been much simpler in his feelings towards her. Not for a moment would he ever have parted with her, any more than with any of the others.

It is because of this that questions about whether you can love two children the same when only one is your own are really impossible to answer, unless you're prepared to be very personal. Because of these special feelings that I have, and my husband also, the 'twins' are equally dear to us. And we love them not only for what they mean to us both, but also for what the two of them mean to each other, and to the whole family. If occasionally I have had regrets that the elder ones were rushed through early childhood a bit too fast, and took maybe too much responsibility, I've realized that all of them have had to fend for themselves also, and all of them seem to thrive on it. It's something I'm proud of. And when Fanny is old enough to realize the implications of having been adopted, it will maybe help her to see and know she isn't different after all: because she'll see that she's had exactly the same as the others, that everything is shared, and that they feel towards her as to each other and that we've always been there for them all.

This is one example of adoptions in this category which emphasizes some of the general points made earlier. The question inevitably arises, however, to what extent adoption by relatives had really served the child's interests. As far as the adopters were concerned, it had given them legal security and legal rights which could not be obtained in any other way. It might be claimed that such benefits were carried over to the children. But the difficulties such adoptions created in the wider family could be counted a high price to pay. For the evidence showed that the effect of granting orders was to confuse relationships—grandparents becoming parents, natural mothers becoming sisters and so forth. The real reason for such applications is that the child may be given the surname of the relatives who are going to bring him up and to give them legal guardianship. It would seem that much more enquiry is needed in order that more flexible legislation can be introduced. Possibly, through amendment to the present guardianship laws, a means of conferring the same security on proxy-parents might be provided, while releasing them and the child from some of the constraints and anxieties implied by adoption.

12

CONCLUSION

SUMMARY

So far the study has been concerned with describing adoption procedure in the survey area, the problems of those responsible for its administration and the reactions of a sample of adoptive parents. The final task is to consider in summary how far, in light of the findings, adoption procedures and practices in general 'protect the three parties concerned from risks which might lead to unhappiness'.[1] Apart from the legal aspects, which are dealt with separately, the four main stages at which protection can at present be given are when the mother decides whether to relinquish or keep her baby; when adopters are selected; when they are matched with a particular child, and finally during the period of supervision which occurs after placement. The main issues and shortcomings at each point are summarized and then discussed more generally.

The Mother's Decision

The Hurst Committee recommended that 'children should be protected from unnecessary separation from their parents' and 'natural parents must be protected from hurried or panic decisions to give up their child, and from being persuaded to place them unsuitably'.[2] The law endeavours to protect mothers from hasty action by requiring them to wait until their baby is six weeks old before they can give a valid consent to adoption. But where parents have little opportunity to discuss their plans for the child

---

[1] Hurst report, p. 4.
[2] Hurst report, p. 4.

with a competent person, the value of this safeguard is reduced. Although natural mothers who relinquished their babies were not interviewed, records and other sources suggested that few had been able to explore the alternatives to adoption in this way. In some cases it appeared doubtful whether alternatives existed which could offer a mother sufficient social and financial provision to enable her to keep her child without considerable difficulty. In particular this seemed likely when she could not, or would not, rely upon the assistance of her family. In the eyes of some natural mothers, even the best alternatives available must have seemed unattractive compared with the advantages the child was assumed to gain from adoption. Carefully considered decisions require real alternatives to choose from, as well as competent and timely assistance.

Selection

Agencies probably have the most effective opportunity to influence the outcome of adoption at the point where they select their applicants. In view of this the general uncertainty which prevailed about selection criteria was disturbing. Whilst all statutory and voluntary agencies agreed that selection was their most important task, there were wide variations in the degree of responsibility taken by committees and officers, in the extent to which trained caseworkers were used, and the amount and type of information collected as a basis for the selection decision. Some agencies spent a good deal of time and took great trouble in getting to know applicants and assessing their offer. In other instances, only very superficial assessments can have been made, since contacts were so limited.

The evidence in the survey suggested that the protection recommended by the Hurst Committee for children from being adopted by 'people unsuited to the responsibility', and for adopters 'from undertaking responsibilities for which they were not fitted, or which they have not appreciated'[1] was not in all cases provided. These instances were not restricted to private adoptions. Where agencies were involved, shortage of trained staff and pressure of work were partly responsible. But more generally there is an

[1] Hurst report, p. 4.

urgent need for research into the whole question of selection, particularly in relation to the eventual outcome of placements. Only in this way can the validity of procedures and criteria be confidently established.

Matching

Once again, although all agencies attached great importance to matching they were unsure what information was relevant. Some of the criteria, as well as being untested, were impossible to apply universally. For instance, in order to match social background, there needs to be roughly equivalent proportions of adopters and children from similar backgrounds: an equivalence which did not exist. The agencies were also hampered by lack of time and opportunity to collect information from natural parents (especially fathers). The applicants, in their turn, were hampered because there was little agreement amongst agencies on the relevance to matching of the applicants' opinions or preferences. In the absence of any follow-up study it is difficult to establish with certainty whether or not the interests of child and adopters were being properly protected at this stage.

Supervision

Statutory supervision, to which all types of adoptions were subject at the time of the survey, should present a further opportunity for protection. From the number of recorded visits however, only limited use had been made of these powers by local authorities; and staff of children's departments were sometimes uncertain about the function of supervision and in particular about what help and advice should or could be given at this stage. Few of the adopters who were interviewed had a clear picture of what supervision was supposed to achieve. Visits had coincided with a time when they were not generally receptive, as they were pre-occupied with the child and with their chance of making him theirs. When advice and support were really needed, when the question of telling the child of his status became pressing, contact with the placing or supervising agency had long been discontinued. Responsibility for telling and for dealing with the consequences weighed heavily on most of the couples seen.

M

As at the other previous stages, it would be very difficult to claim that the welfare of child and adopters was adequately protected at this time. Contact was brief, and objectives and scope insufficiently clear to both child care staff and applicants.

DISCUSSION

General Problems

It seemed that present safeguards were inadequate in many respects. However, the problem of securing better help and protection for all three parties must be seen against the general background of a number of major issues. One problem which has continually reappeared throughout the study is the disparity between the number of people who wish to adopt and the babies or children available. This had repercussions on the work of adoption agencies (particularly at the stage of selection) and thus upon the service that many adopters received. In many cases this difficulty was aggravated by a widely acknowledged lack of sufficient staff, particularly trained staff. The problem of selection, for instance, seems to dominate the work of adoption agencies, and unless existing staff are not to be overwhelmed by the task of interviewing most of their applicants sympathetically and skilfully, somewhat arbitrary rules of eligibility must be expected. These serve to reduce the work load and may allow more time and attention to be paid to those applicants who can satisfy them. In general, the adoption societies seemed anxious to use reliable and justifiable rules whereby some applications could be rejected outright. Unfortunately, as many of them admitted, there is no evidence from which to judge reliability, although some justification might be claimed for restrictions like those about the maximum age of adopters. One repercussion of the use of such rules of initial eligibility seemed to be that applicants could be rejected with insufficient regard for their needs and feelings. Adopters who had experienced rejection certainly complained of this.

If more trained staff were recruited the problem would probably become less acute. Were there a large infusion, more time could be spent on selection as well as matching and supervision, and better decisions probably made. The gap between demand and supply however would remain unaffected and would continue to influence the work, particularly as it seems more likely to widen than close. If, for instance, the recommendation made by many of the adopters for more information and publicity led to action, this would hardly reduce demand. Likewise better counselling services and information for unmarried mothers, together with improved facilities, may well encourage and enable them to keep, rather than surrender their babies. More illegitimate births will probably be offset by the growing popularity of marriage which presumably increases, at least proportionately, the number of couples wishing to adopt. Of course we do not know the size of the potential demand for adoption: applicants often apply to several agencies simultaneously and there is little information about the incidence of sterility or infertility. Nevertheless, any potential demand is more likely to become explicit in the atmosphere of greater public sympathy and tolerance of adoption; which many adopters hoped would gradually emerge. In the same way less censorious attitudes to illegitimacy may encourage more unmarried mothers to keep their babies.

Thus the gap between supply and demand is likely to remain a characteristic feature of adoption and a major problem all agencies will continue to face. However, more and better trained staff can probably ensure first that a minimum, and then that a higher standard of service is offered. Are there particular forms of administration which will enable the adoption services to mobilize more resources, in particular manpower? It would appear that small organizations, already drastically understaffed, are in the weakest position. In contrast, larger organizations, particularly those in process of growing, will be in a stronger position to attract additional resources. From the previous discussion it seems unlikely that agencies with only adoption functions will have a great deal of scope for growth. This will be more likely to occur in organizations with a multi-purpose basis. In light of the developments in the field of prevention, introduced in the 1963 Children and Young Persons Act, and the recent White Paper[1] canvassing the possibilities of a family service, growth is most likely to occur in the local authority children's departments. In the writer's opinion, the most desirable move would be an

[1] *The Child, the Family and the Young Offender*, Cmnd. 2742, 1965.

immediate enquiry to find out why some local authorities have not yet made use of their permissive powers conferred by the Adoption Act 1958 which allows them to arrange the adoption of children not actually in their care. The sheer volume of orders granted annually must alone mean that adoption has now reached the proportions of a public service. As such the service ought to be provided everywhere by public as well as by private agencies.[1] Already by 1958 in the study area the children's departments had been able to recruit a significantly greater proportion of trained staff than any of the adoption societies. Adoption work had, it seemed, gained almost incidentally from general improvements in other aspects of their work, since the child care staff undertook a variety of duties.

In other respects the future of the single function agencies, those that only place children for adoption but accept no responsibility for helping the mother to take her decision or for supervision, might be questioned. Today more is understood about the shortcomings that ensue when complex problems are tackled piecemeal without sufficient regard for their context. No one would claim for instance, that the unmarried mother's needs are met satisfactorily merely by planning her child's adoption. Since the local authorities already have statutory duties to supervise adoption placements and are frequently involved as *guardian ad litem*, the more a unified service for all parties is considered desirable, the more likely are they to increase and improve their adoption functions.

In general the clues in this study point to the social value of multi-purpose agencies, organizing and providing a wide range of related services of which all the parties to adoption may stand in need. The provision of an easily accessible counselling service staffed by professional social workers; the availability of alternative forms of help for the natural mothers (like nurseries, foster homes, or specially reserved accommodation) are amongst the services which might compose an efficient and comprehensive organization. Indeed the results of this study would lend support to the idea of such provision forming part of an emerging family

[1] By November 1965, 74 of the 171 counties and county boroughs in England and Wales were acting as adoption agencies. (Personal communication, Children's Department, Home Office).

service rather than developing farther as a highly specialized field. If this occurred several advantages would seem to accrue to mothers, children, adopters, and the service.

For the natural parents help would not be limited only to planning for their child. The alternatives to adoption would be explored and implemented with the agencies' help if need be. The parents would have the comfort of knowing that the same agency (and perhaps the same official) would be involved throughout. If they decided to part with their child this could be planned in accordance with their readiness and not, as is sometimes now the case, in accordance with the availability of a home. The agency would be certain to accept responsibility for the child (unlike the present practice of some societies) even if the child was later found not to be suitable for adoption. Contact with the parents could be maintained as long as desired.

For the child the paramount advantage would be that there was greater assurance than at present that he was not needlessly deprived of his natural parents' care. Decisions would more likely be based on timely, comprehensive planning, and a full range of services could be exploited in his interests.

Adopters in their turn could depend on the advice and support of trained staff able to offer at least a basic minimum standard of service. Matching could be undertaken by a worker who knew all three parties and supervision would be the continuation of the process begun at selection. Once adoption was regarded as one of many services offered by the general welfare agency, adopters would probably feel less conspicuous about seeking help in the post-adoption period. There would be advantage in that the agency that had established initial contact would be at hand.

The advantages of a family service would probably have a bearing on staffing too, since it could be held that the narrower the range of problems, the greater the strain on the staff. Family agencies would offer facilities for a wide range of work, and career prospects in general would probably seem to be more attractive. The possibility of promotion in social work generally, rather than the particular field of adoption, would clearly be enhanced. From the practical aspect various grades of staff could be deployed to the best advantage: the most highly skilled could act as supervisors and consultants to the less experienced and newly-trained; an important point in view of the back log of untrained personnel whose services will inevitably continue to be needed for many years. In brief, the larger family service organization would enable adoption work to share in certain common facilities (like consultations) which in many instances they are at present denied.

The Legal Aspects

As well as changes in administrative structure, the fuller use of existing legal provisions and also changes in the law might help to raise standards. More use, for example, might be made of the regulations governing the statutory registration of voluntary societies by the local authorities in whose area their headquarters are located. These regulations include amongst their provisions that a local authority shall refuse to register an adoption society if the number of competent persons employed is, in the opinion of the authority, insufficient, having regard to the extent of the activities.[1] At the moment the potential value of the registration system seems lost. Judging by the comments of children's officers, little more generally than the collection of statistical returns seems at present to be involved. Yet registration is one of the few tools specifically designed to assess, enforce and raise a minimum standard of service. As long ago as 1937, the conditions for registration at present in force were set out; and it was pointed out that registration confers a certain prestige and tends to be regarded by the public as a hall-mark of approval.[2] No code is sufficient without inspection, and inspection without enforcement is useless. Children's officers seem to regard the task of acting as inspectors to their voluntary society colleagues as invidious. And anyway, as they themselves begin to act as placement agencies they too should be subject to inspection. This suggests that inspection should become a task of central government rather than local government. Although the Home Office undertakes periodical reviews of all the other aspects of each children's department's work, the sphere of adoption is still left out.

Statutory supervision of placements might also be used more

[1] Adoption Act, 1958, Section 30.
[2] Report of the Departmental Committee on Adoption Societies and Agencies, 1937, Cmd. 5499, p. 44.

fully and perhaps modified. The evidence in this enquiry suggests room for further use and this might be assured by legally prescribing a minimum number of visits. The present regulations merely stipulate that a visit must be paid within a month of the placement. If the aims of supervision are seen more broadly as helping the integration of the new family, a longer period than the present three months would seem appropriate. This would be a difficult move (and unpopular with the adopters) without provisions being made whereby natural parents who so wish can relinquish their parental rights to the agency within a given period of placing their child in its care for adoption. Such a system has found favour in several parts of Canada and the United States. Were such measures introduced here, applicants could be relieved of the fear that at the eleventh hour their child might be 'snatched back'. Freed from this anxiety they would probably be more receptive during the period of supervision. This period could then be extended, if necessary, without either applicants or agency feeling that there was a desperate need to hurry on to the hearing. Such possibilities of natural parents relinquishing their child to an agency would remove a major criticism of the potentially valuable system of 'fostering with a view to adoption'.

Such a change in law would also promote the child's interest. The danger of his being uprooted would be reduced, for the removal of obstacles to his surrender would tend to sponsor earlier and final relinquishment. This legal amendment presupposes the adequate provision of a casework service, to help all parents who need assistance to reach their decision as soon as possible after the child's birth. Unfortunately such provisions cannot as yet be described as adequate.

Equally, this proposed change probably represents a more desirable approach to the natural parents' problem. Surely, to reach and to stand by this difficult decision they should be given every possible assistance? Were the voluntary termination of parental rights to be made possible, no further consent to adoption would be required. This would avoid the present difficult situation which arises whenever delay in adoption occurs: in such cases, months or years after mother and child have gone their separate ways, the guardian has to seek out the mother on the court's behalf, to verify her views and her consent. Such legal amendment would tie in with the recommendation that the needs of parent and child should always be met by one and the same agency.

In connection with the legal aspects of adoption by relatives, one point to query is how far welfare is promoted by the recent change in law whereby, if one of the applicants is a natural parent, they need no longer give the local authority three months' notice of their intention to adopt. This category of children does not fall within the 'protected child' category. Local authorities seem generally to have interpreted this change as exempting them from 'welfare authority' responsibility; their contact now being restricted to *guardian ad litem* duties—where the children's officer is so appointed. The writer found that these adopters' need for the help and advice of a trained caseworker was at least as great as that of any of the other categories. Often it was they who had had to make the most difficult and subtle adjustments. Where relatives other than the natural parents look after a child, a modified form of legal guardianship might provide a more suitable alternative: for by its nature adoption imposes an artificial stamp on the pattern of family relationships, which could have undesirable consequences for all the members of the family.

Direct private placements are not subjected to the same safeguards provided in the case of third party adoptions. No notice to the local authority need be given in the case of children placed by their mothers and amendment to the law in this respect seems desirable. Third party and private placements are likely to continue but ought to be adequately safeguarded. In order to supplement the very tenuous benefits of the 'notice of placement' system, parents proposing to place their child for adoption might be required to satisfy a competent body that they had fully explored the alternatives and that their proposed plans were the best that could be made for the child in all the circumstances.

Finally, there is the small but important problem of children in respect of whom an adoption order has been refused. Twenty years ago, it was recommended that where applications were refused because the home was unsuitable, the court should be empowered to commit the child to the care of a local authority.

The need to establish a sufficient case against the applicants in court has made it exceedingly difficult for local authorities to take action. Hence, children placed unsuitably may yet remain where they are. This is another problem calling for further investigation in order that the spirit of the legislation can be enacted.

Even where children are adopted by relatives, making the order should not be merely a matter of rubber stamping a legal transaction. But courts do give the impression that they frequently have little concern with anything but the legal aspects of adoption. This impression, as well as reports of the speed with which hearings were often despatched, the premises in which applications were heard, and the fact that the final decision was taken by people with a lay or essentially legal background, suggest that thought should be given to how adoption cases are heard and by whom. It has been suggested that the family courts proposed by the recent White Paper[1] should deal with adoption. This would remove them from the atmosphere of criminal proceedings and if those serving these courts were well chosen, in having a broad range of training and experience, they might deal better with the complex legal, social and emotional questions relevant to adoption applications. Such changes would receive the warm support of most of the adopters interviewed in this study.

The Need for Publicity and Literature

The lack of publicity and of specially designed adoption literature has an adverse effect on all three parties to adoption. For example, the advantages of agency-sponsored adoptions ought to be better known, and it is regrettable that agencies hide their light under a bushel. Whatever the individual failings of agencies, the placements they arrange have clear advantages over those arranged by inexperienced people. Private or third party placements may be agreed when neither natural or adoptive parents are fully aware of the risks to them and the child. Clear, concise and readily available literature setting out community resources and the pros and cons of different forms of proceeding to adoption would be invaluable to those anticipating parting

[1] Ibid., p. 9.

with their child. There is also a need for literature aimed at those who share in arranging private placements, particularly members of the medical profession. The law on third party adoption should be better advertised, partly through the prosecution of defaulters.

Many adopters regretted the absence of means of informing themselves in advance of applying to adopt. They wanted general information as well as help in distinguishing between the various ways of adopting and between the various requirements of different agencies. Such information and help might take the form of literature, but additionally it could be supplied by the development of group meetings for prospective adopters before application. These have been developed by some agencies in North America and the recently established British Adoption Project is also employing this approach. At such meetings a dozen couples might be invited to hear of the agencies' policies, principles and practices and general discussion encouraged. Those who decide to pursue their application to adopt can then proceed in the normal way. This development would not only serve the purpose of providing information and opportunity for discussion, but might be a means of conserving the time of the staff available. Group meetings would also reduce the number of applicants who are at present rejected outright as ineligible.

Many adopters felt that community attitudes towards adopters and adopted children left something to be desired: many had encountered ignorance and prejudice, which was partly ascribed to the lack of literature. If the climate of opinion is not sufficiently favourable, conflicts for adopters and child may result which could undermine even the best of placements.

Further Research

Whatever changes occur in the organization and staffing of the adoption services, and whatever legal modifications might be introduced, there remains the fact that remarkably little is known about adoption: particularly the outcome of adoption. For instance, which sorts of couples make the best adopters, and anyway what is 'best'? There is often no opportunity for individual social workers to observe how their selection decisions work out, and since systematic follow-up studies have not been undertaken, there is little possibility of building up a reliable body of know-ledge from past experience. The call for more trained staff is laudable, but can the training they receive include such reliable knowledge based upon past experience? If anything, it was the trained staff who in this study voiced the greatest doubts about their decisions: the untrained were more confident in their common-sense approach.

Many problems and much of the uncertainty highlighted in this report might be reduced by the increased knowledge that research could provide. There are no signs that co-operation would not be forthcoming. The adopters in this enquiry were not merely pleased but even relieved to participate, and the refusal rate was low. Agencies were equally interested and ready to take part. They recognized that research was a means of improving practice, and that better use needed to be made of accumulated experience if skills were to be refined.

So much needs to be done that some indication of priorities is required. Voluntary and statutory agencies might jointly draw up a research programme and confer on priorities, confidentiality, and the general problems of getting research discussed, accepted and acted upon. If agencies began by examining their basic recording systems with a view to designing a uniform minimum standard, subsequent research could start from a firmer foundation.

There are many difficulties to be faced if adequate follow-up studies are to be made, whether they be concerned with special groups (such as the mentally subnormal, the older child, the privately placed child, or mothers adopting their own children) or particular decisions (about selection, rejection, making interim orders and so forth). One difficulty is getting sufficient research resources, but another, closely related, is the need to develop comparative studies. Essentially the dilemma in adoption is not restricted to whether a child should go to these applicants or those, but includes the question whether another form of care altogether might serve the child better. Ideally a wide range of comparative follow-up studies is required. For instance, comparisons ought to be made between children kept by their unmarried mothers and those relinquished for adoption; between couples accepted as adopters and those rejected; between adoptive families and foster families. And so the list could continue.

Although the greatest need is clearly for a variety of follow-up studies and the evaluation of decisions, much might be achieved by smaller and less ambitious research, merely aiming to collect data or describe what is happening. How, for instance, do the adopters who proceed privately differ from those helped by an agency? The straightforward collection of information, particularly about the natural parents, would be valuable. At the moment details of the natural fathers are conspicuous by their absence and much more also needs to be known about the mothers. What, for example, distinguishes those who relinquish their babies from those who keep them?[1] Without basic information such as this it is difficult to plan an adequate adoption service and make appropriate decisions about selection and matching.

This study looked at the views and opinions, problems and aspirations of a small group of adopters. Similar descriptive studies, or others focusing more upon the natural mothers, might be undertaken elsewhere. It would indeed be valuable to approach this same group again some years hence, to see what new problems had arisen, what old ones had disappeared and how they had been overcome.

Hitherto, the lack of sponsorship, shortage of staff, time and funds, and fears about confidentiality have all contributed to the neglect of adoption research in this country. But in view of what is at stake, and confronted by the abysmal ignorance which clouds every issue, can we any longer afford not to provide resources for research? The writer, and it is hoped the reader, is in no doubt as to the immense scope and absolute necessity for action.

---

[1] See, for example, Margaret Yelloly, *Factors Relating to an Adoption Decision by the Mothers of Illegitimate Infants*. The Sociological Review, Vol. 13, No. 1 (New Series), March 1965.

APPENDIX 1

THE following is a copy of the letter sent out by the children's officer on the department's official notepaper. Each was individually typed and marked, 'Private and Confidential'.

Dear Mr and Mrs . . . . . .
An adoption survey is being carried out by a former child welfare worker, Mrs Iris Goodacre, and I am writing to ask whether you may be willing to take part.

Those who have already adopted a child can be of great help to future adopters, to children's departments, the courts, and to all those concerned with the welfare of children, because they have personal experience to pass on. You could assist, by letting the research worker have comments on the arrangements made for your child's adoption.*

I do assure you that this survey is entirely confidential. Neither the families taking part, nor even the counties in which they live, will be identifiable in the report on the enquiry. The research worker will visit by appointment only, at any time convenient to you. She would not, of course, interview anyone but yourselves, unless with your express consent.

Should you state that you do not wish to take part, you will not hear anything further. However, as your experience could be most useful in promoting the happiness of the many children still to be adopted, I do hope you will allow Mrs Goodacre to call on you, to tell you herself about this important enquiry.

You are asked to complete the form attached to this letter, and I enclose a stamped, addressed envelope for your reply. If you would be kind enough to let me have this back as soon as possible, I should be most grateful.

Yours sincerely,
. . . .
Children's Officer.

The reply form enclosed with all letters offered these alternatives . . .

(1) We are willing for the research worker to call
on . . . . . . day, the . . . . of . . . .(month)
at . . . . o'clock.
or:
(2) We do not wish to take part in the survey.

Signed . . . .
address . . . .

N

Mothers adopting their own illegitimate child following first marriage were sent identical letters, with the exception that an extra paragraph was inserted at the point marked*. This was introduced as a result of the experience gained during the course of the pilot survey, when these adopters had frequently commented that 'their kind of adoption' could not possibly be relevant to the survey. To forestall such reactions, the following lines were added to the letter they received:

'It may interest you to know that almost half of all adoption orders granted concern children who are related to one of the adopters. Because adoptions by mothers and their husbands of children born before marriage occur so often, this group of adopters can give specially valuable information to the research worker; for they can comment on the services given to the unmarried mother, and on their experience following marriage.'

APPENDIX 2

THE LEGAL BACKGROUND

THE two main objects in this appendix are to sketch in the law relating to adopters, to natural parents and to the child, and to give an abstract of local authority, agency and court procedure in relation to adoption practice. The summary deals only with those portions of the law most relevant to the foregoing discussion. Extensive reference is made to the Adoption Act 1958, the Adoption (Juvenile Court) Rules 1959 (which differ in certain respects from the High Court and County Court Rules), and to the summary of the Adoption Act given in the Home Office *Eighth Report on the Work of the Children's Department, 1961.* Some wording is taken verbatim from each of the above sources, but inverted commas are mostly omitted to simplify the presentation.

For an exposition of the law, reference must of course be made to the statutes currently in force—as well as to recent case law. The earlier Adoption Acts and Committees of Enquiry, which led to and resulted from changes in legislation are also of great interest, particularly the first Adoption Act of 1926, the Report of the Departmental Committee on Adoption Societies and Agencies 1937 (the 'Horsbrugh' Report) and the Report of the Departmental Committee on the Adoption of Children, 1954 (the Hurst Report) which led to the latest changes in adoption law.

What is *the effect of making an adoption order?* On an order being made, all rights, duties, obligations and liabilities of the parents or guardians of the infant in relation to future custody, maintenance and education shall be extinguished, and all such rights, duties, obligations and liabilities shall vest in and be exercisable by and enforceable against the adopters as if the infant were a child born to the adopters in lawful wedlock.[1] In relation to marriage, the adopters and the person whom they have been authorized to adopt are deemed to be within the prohibited degrees of consanguinity. If the adopter, the adopted person or anyone else dies intestate, any property devolves as if the adopted person were the child of the adopter born in lawful wedlock.[2] An infant who is not a citizen of the United Kingdom and Colonies becomes such a citizen from the date of the order if the adopter, or the male adopter is of British nationality.[3]

Only 'infants' may be adopted. An 'infant' is defined as a person under the age of 21 years, but the definition does not include a person who is or has

---

[1] Adoption Act, 1958, Section 13.
[2] Ibid., Section 16.
[3] Adoption Act, 1958, Section 19.

been married.[1] An adoption order cannot be made in England and Wales unless both the applicant and the 'infant' are domiciled in England and Wales. Provisional adoption orders, however, may now be granted to persons not ordinarily domiciled in this country.[2]

Who may make orders? An application may be made to the High Court or, at the option of the applicants, to any county court or juvenile court within the jurisdiction of which the applicant or infant reside at the date of the application.[3]

There are some *restrictions on making adoption arrangements*. Subject to certain conditions, there is no restriction on an individual making adoption arrangements; but no body of persons may make such arrangements unless it is a registered adoption society or a local authority.[4] Local authorities may participate whether or not the child for whom certain arrangements are to be made is in their care.[5] Payments, or promises, of payment or reward, in consideration of adoption arrangements are not lawful except as sanctioned by the court.[6] Restrictions on advertising make it unlawful to advertise that a parent desires an infant to be adopted, that a person desires to adopt, or that a person is willing to make adoption arrangements.[7]

Who may adopt? An order may be made on the application of two spouses authorizing them jointly to adopt an infant, but in no other case can more than one person adopt an infant.[8] The adoption of an infant by his mother or father, either alone or jointly with his or her spouse, is authorized.[9] An order cannot be made unless (*a*) the applicant is the mother or father of the infant; (*b*) is a relative of the infant and has attained the age of 21, or (*c*) has attained the age of 25. In the case of joint applicants other than the mother or father, one applicant must have reached the age of 25, and the other attained the age of 21 years. A female child cannot be adopted by a sole male applicant unless the court is satisfied that such an exceptional measure is justified.[10]

Procedure. Before an adoption order can be made the infant must have been continuously in the care of the applicant for at least three consecutive months preceding the date of the order, not counting any time before the child is six weeks old.[11] Unless the applicant or one of the applicants is a parent of the infant, or the infant has reached school leaving age by the date of the hearing, the applicant must notify the local authority in writing of his intention to apply for an adoption order at least three months before an order can be made.[11]

[1] Ibid., Section 57.
[2] Ibid., Section 1.
[3] Ibid., Section 12.
[4] Ibid., Section 9.
[5] Ibid., Section 29.
[6] Ibid., Section 28.
[7] Ibid., Section 50.
[8] Ibid., Section 51.
[9] Ibid., Section 1.
[10] Adoption Act, 1958, Section 2.
[11] Ibid., Section 3.

Receipt of this written notification (the 'statutory notification') by the local authority means that the infant becomes a 'protected' child.[1] The local authority then has the duty to visit 'from time to time' until the order is made or until he reaches the age of 18, whichever occurs first. Local authority officers must satisfy themselves as to the well-being of protected children and give such advice as to their care and maintenance 'as may appear to be needed'.[2]

Local authority officers are authorized to inspect any premises in their area in which such 'protected' children are to be or are being kept.[3] Refusal to allow a 'protected 'child to be visited by an authorized officer is a punishable offence.[4]

While an application for an order is pending in any court (i.e. after the applicants have given the local authority written notification of their intention to apply for an adoption order) a parent who has signified his consent may not—except with leave of the court—remove the infant from the applicants. In considering whether to grant or refuse such leave, the court must have regard to the welfare of the infant.[5] There are restrictions on the return of infants placed either by adoption societies or local authorities, neither of whom may remove a child placed for adoption except with leave of the court, once an application has been made.[6] There is no time limit within which the person with whom the infant is placed must either apply for an order or return the infant. But if an infant has been placed by a society or local authority and the person with whom the infant has been placed withdraws his application, then the infant must be returned within seven days to the society or authority. At any time before an order has been made, an applicant can give notice of his intention not to retain the infant.[7]

As soon as practicable after an application has been made the court *appoints* some person to act as the *guardian ad litem* of the infant with the duty of safeguarding the interests of the infant before the court.[8] The Adoption (Juvenile Court) Rules 1959 makes provision concerning the person appointed, and define his duties. The guardian must be the childen's officer of a local authority or a member of his staff, providing the local authority consents, or else a probation officer, unless exceptionally the court considers it is impracticable or undesirable in the particular case to appoint any of these persons. Apart from safeguarding the interests of the infant, it is the guardian's duty 'to investigate all circumstances relevant to the proposed adoption, including the matters alleged in the application' and to make a confidential report in writing to the court. No person can be appointed guardian if he

[1] Ibid., Section 37.
[2] Ibid., Section 38.
[3] Ibid., Section 39.
[4] Ibid., Section 44.
[5] Ibid., Section 35.
[6] Ibid., Section 36.
[7] Adoption Act, 1958, Section 35.
[8] Ibid., Section 9.

has rights as a parent of the infant, has taken part in the arrangements for the infant's adoption, or is an official of a local authority or adoption society that has taken part in the arrangements for that child's adoption. At the time of appointing the guardian, the court must fix a time for the hearing of the application.

The *'Particular Duties of the Guardian ad Litem'*[1] include that he must interview the applicant, ascertain particulars of all members of the applicant's household, of the accommodation and condition of the home, the applicant's means, his state of health, whether the referee he has nominated is a responsible person and recommends the applicant, and whether the applicant understands the nature of an adoption order and, in particular that he understands 'the order, if made, will render him responsible for the maintenance and upbringing of the infant'.

The guardian must ascertain whether the infant is able to understand the nature of an adoption order, and if so, whether he wishes to be adopted by the applicant. The *guardian ad litem* must interview, or appoint an agent to interview, every individual who is a respondent to the application, and every individual who appears to him to have taken part in the arrangements for the child's adoption. The guardian must obtain from every respondent not being an individual (i.e. an adoption agency or local authority) such information concerning the infant as they consider might assist the court in deciding whether or not the infant should be adopted by the applicant. The guardian must ascertain when the infant's mother ceased to have care and possession of him; to whom care and possession was transferred; and that every consent to the making of an order is freely given and with full understanding of its nature.

Where an infant is illegitimate but no one is liable as the putative father to contribute to his maintenance, the guardian must inform the court if he learns of any person claiming to be the father, or of any other person who wishes or who ought, in the guardian's opinion, to be heard by the court on the question whether an adoption order should be made.

The court's functions as to adoption orders include that before making an adoption order, the court shall be satisfied that every person whose consent is necessary, and whose consent is not dispensed with, has consented to and understands the nature and effect of the adoption order 'and in particular in the case of any parent, understands that the effect of the order will be permanently to deprive him or her of his or her parental rights'; 'that the order if made will be for the welfare of the infant'; and that no payment or other reward has been made, given or agreed. In determining whether an adoption order will be for the infant's welfare, the court shall have regard (among other things) to the health of the applicant and the wishes of the infant.[2]

An adoption order may not be made except with the consent of every person who is a parent or guardian of the infant; nor can it be made on the

[1] The Adoption (Juvenile Court) Rules, 1959, Second Schedule.
[2] Adoption Act, 1958, Section 7.

application of one of two spouses, unless the other spouse also consents. The consent of a natural father is not required, nor that of any person who is liable or has agreed to contribute to the maintenance of the infant.[1] The mother may not give her consent in law, until the child is at least six weeks old.[2] The court has power to dispense with any consent if, amongst other reasons it is satisfied that the person whose consent is to be dispensed with has abandoned, neglected or persistently ill treated the infant; or cannot be found or is incapable of giving his consent or is withholding his consent unreasonably; or has persistently failed without reasonable cause to discharge the obligations of a parent or guardian of the infant. If a person who has consented without knowing the identity of the applicant subsequently withdraws his consent only because he does not know the identity of the applicant, his consent shall be deemed to be unreasonably withheld.[3] A person proposing to apply for an adoption order and wishing to keep his identity confidential may obtain in advance of his application a serial number and the form of consent will then identify the applicant by the serial number only.[4] If a serial number has been assigned, the proceedings are to be so conducted that the applicant is not seen by, or made known to any respondent not already aware of his identity—except with his consent.[5]

Every application is heard and determined *in camera*.[6] The Rules provide that the court shall not make any adoption order except after the personal attendance before the court of the applicants.[7] Respondents may attend the proceedings for the purpose of giving their consents, but written evidence of their consent is admissible as evidence provided the documents are properly attested.[8] The court may postpone the determination of the application and make an interim order, giving custody of the infant to the applicants for not more than two years by way of a probationary period.[9]

When the court has made its decision, the clerk serves notice of the effect on all parties who were not present at the time.[10] If an order or interim order has been made, an abridged copy must be served on the applicant and if it is a full order, a copy must be sent to the Registrar General.[11] The copy of the order which the applicant receives contains entries giving the date and county of the child's birth, the Registration District and sub-district, the name, surname and sex of the infant; the name, surname, address and occupation of the adopter or adopters; and the date of the adoption order and

---

[1] Ibid., Section 4.
[2] Ibid., Section 6.
[3] Adoption Act, 1958, Section 5.
[4] The Adoption (Juvenile Court) Rules 1959, clause 2.
[5] Ibid., clause 15.
[6] Ibid., clause 16.
[7] Ibid., clause 13.
[8] Adoption Act, 1958, Section 6.
[9] Ibid., Section 8.
[10] Adoption (Juvenile Court) Rules, 1959, clause 25.
[11] Ibid., clause 27.

description of the court by which it was made.[1] Every adoption order requires entries to be made in the Adopted Children Register, which enable the Registrar-General in most cases to issue a certificate similar to the shortened form of the birth certificate.[2] (The equivalent to the 'long' birth certificate for an adopted child is a copy of the Adoption order in which the parents are described as adopters.) Every person is entitled to search the Adopted Children Register, kept in the General Registrar Office. In addition to this register, the Registrar keeps such other registers as may be necessary to record and make traceable the connection between entries in the Register of Births and corresponding entries in the Adopted Children Register. In England and Wales these other registers are not open to public inspection or search except under a court order.[2] (This is one of several provisions which distinguish English from Scottish adoption legislation.)

Certain provisions specifically relate to adoptive applicants who are either the *infant's mother or father*. For example, in these cases no medical certificate as to the health of the applicants is required, and they need not give three months' notice of their intention to adopt to the local authority.

Where *'third party' adoptions* are concerned (i.e. those arranged by an individual, and not by a registered agency or local authority) the most important provision is that notice of the proposed placement must be given to the local authority by the person who is arranging the infant's transfer. No such notice need be given by the infant's parent or guardinan, or by the person receiving the child in the event of a direct placement. But where a child is placed by an intermediary (unless in an emergency) a local authority must be given at least two week's notice of a proposed placement. Failure to give this required notice is an offence, punishable by a term of imprisonment not exceeding six months, a fine not exceeding £100, or both. If the local authority thinks it would be detrimental to a child to be so placed, it can prohibit the person from receiving the child. Likewise, on the complaint of a local authority, if a Magistrates court feels a 'protected' child is being kept, or is about to be received by a person unfit to have his care, it can make an order to remove the child to a place of safety.

---

[1] See 'Schedule' to The Adoption (Juvenile Court) Rules 1959.
[2] The Adoption Act 1958, Section 20.

—————

ADDITIONAL STATISTICS[1]

SOME of the statistics derived from a study of the files have been included in the main text as tables or in passing reference. It was thought valuable to set out some of the others systematically in an appendix. Each type of adoption has been numbered for ease of presentation. Category I are mothers adopting their own children; category II local authority placements; category III adoption society placements; category IV private placements, and category V adoptions undertaken by relatives.

1. *The Natural Mothers*

TABLE (1)
Natural mother's age at child's birth analysed by adoption categories

	Cat. I		Cat. II		Cat. III		Cat. IV		Cat. V		Total	
	No.	%	No.	%	No.	%	No.	%	No.	%	No.	%
Under 18	8	8	10	14	15	21	1	4	3	11	37	12
18 under 20	20	20	13	18	14	20	–	–	7	26	54	18
20 under 25	42	41	22	30	19	27	14	64	5	19	102	35
25 under 30	21	20	14	19	11	15	3	14	4	14	53	18
30 under 35	7	7	5	7	6	8	4	18	–	–	22	8
35 and over	2	2	4	5	2	3	–	–	3	11	11	4
No information	2	2	5	7	4	6	–	–	5	19	16	5
	102	100	73	100	71	100	22	100	27	100	295	100
Median Ages in yrs.	22·6		22·5		21·2		24·3		21·0		22·4	

[1] Certain other statistical material was collected as well as this offered in the appendix. This can be made available upon application to the National Institute for Social Work Training.

TABLE (II)

Natural mother's other children at birth of the adopted child analysed by categories

	Cat. I		Cat. II		Cat. III		Cat. IV		Cat. V		Total	
	No.	%	No.	%	No.	%	No.	%	No.	%	No.	%
None	82	80	29	40	57	80	8	36	17	63	193	65
One legitimate	10		8		3		2		2		25	
Two or more legitimate	3	13	14	30	3	9	4	28	6	29	30	19
One illegitimate	4		17		7		4		1		33	
Two or more illegitimate	2	6	8	34		10	4	36	–	4	14	16
One legitimate, but not husband's:	–	–	4		1	1	–	–	–	–	5	
Two or more legitimate but not husband's	1	1	2	8	–		–		–		3	3
No information	–	–	1	1	–	–	–	–	1	4	2	1
	102	100	73*	100*	71	100	22	100	27	100	295	100*

2. The Children

TABLE (III)

Adopted child's age at placement analysed by the categories

	Cat. I		Cat. II		Cat. III		Cat. IV		Cat. V		Total	
	No.	%	No.	%	No.	%	No.	%	No.	%	No.	%
Under 6 months	8	8	36	49	57	81	18	81	20	74	139	47
6 months under 1 year	5	5	17	23	10	14	2	9	–	–	34	12
1 year under 2 years	21	20	9	12	2	3	1	5	–	–	33	11
2 years under 3 years	21	20	5	7	1	1	–	–	1	4	28	10
3 years under 5 years	19	19	4	6	–	–	–	–	3	11	26	9
5 years under 10 years	16	16	2	3	1	1	1	5	1	4	21	7
10 years and over	11	11	–	–	–	–	–	–	2	7	13	4
No information	1	1	–	–	–	–	–	–	–	–	1	–
	102	100	73	100	71	100	22	100	27	100	295	100
Median Ages in yrs.	2·7		0·5		0·3		0·3		0·3		0·6	

(*Double counting occurs because classes are not exclusive).

TABLE (IV)

Child's legal status analysed by categories

	Cat. I		Cat. II		Cat. III		Cat. IV		Cat. V		Total	
	No.	%	No.	%	No.	%	No.	%	No.	%	No.	%
Legitimate	25	24	9	12	–	–	2	9	10	37	46	16
Illegitimate	61	60	50	69	62	87	16	73	14	52	203	68
Legitimate but not husband's	16	16	14	19	9	13	4	18	3	11	46	16
	102	100	73	100	71	100	22	100	27	100	295	100

3. *Adopters*

TABLE (V)

The age of the adoptive mother at placement analysed by adoption categories

	Cat. I		Cat. II		Cat. III		Cat. IV		Cat. V		Total	
	No.	%	No.	%	No.	%	No.	%	No.	%	No.	%
Under 20	27	27	–	–	–	–	–	–	–	–	27	9
20 under 25	41	40	6	8	1	1	–	–	2	7	50	17
25 under 30	25	24	23	31	16	23	5	23	1	4	70	24
30 under 35	8	8	16	22	26	37	6	27	5	18	61	21
35 under 40	1	1	18	25	17	24	2	9	4	15	42	14
40 under 50	–	–	10	14	11	15	9	41	12	44	42	14
50 and over	–	–	–	–	–	–	–	–	1	4	1	–
No information	–	–	–	–	–	–	–	–	1	4	1	} 1
Not applicable	–	–	–	–	–	–	–	–	1	4	1	
	102	100	73	100	71	100	22	100	27	100	295	100
Median Age in Yrs.	22·9		32·3		33·4		35·0		40·4		30·0	

TABLE (VI)

Number of years adoptive parents married analysed by categories

	Cat. I		Cat. II		Cat. III		Cat. IV		Cat. V		Total	
	No.	%	No.	%	No.	%	No.	%	No.	%	No.	%
Under 2 years	52	51	–	–	1	1	1	5	–	–	54	18
2 years under 6 years	31	30	10	14	11	16	6	27	3	11	61	21
6 years under 10 years	10	10	23	31	29	41	11	50	7	26	80	27
10 years or more	9	9	31	43	30	42	4	18	16	59	90	31
No information/ not applicable	–	–	9	12	–	–	–	–	1	4	10	3
	102	100	73	100	71	100	22	100	27	100	295	100

Table (VII)

Structure of adopters' families at placement analysed by categories

	Cat. I		Cat. II		Cat. III		Cat. IV		Cat. V		Total	
	No.	%	No.	%	No.	%	No.	%	No.	%	No.	%
No children	68	67	42	58	42	59	12	54	11	41	175	59
Own or Step children	34	33	17	23	13	18	7	32	13	48	84	28
Adopted children	–	–	12	16	18	25	4	18	4	15	38	13
No information	–	–	2	3	–	–	–	–	–	–	2	1
	102	100	73	100	71*	100	22*	100	27*	100	295*	100

(*Double counting occurs because classes are not exclusive).

(Table VIII)

Ages of adopted children at the time of survey visit

	Cat. I	Cat. II	Cat. III	Cat. IV	Cat. V	Total
Under 5	–	5	8	8	4	24
5 under 8	3	11	14	8	6	41
8 under 11	9	6	–	–	1	16
11 and over	6	1	1	–	5	13
	18	23	23	16	16	94

BIBLIOGRAPHY

Official publications
Report of the Committee on Child Adoption, Cmd. 1254, 1921.
Departmental Committee on Adoption Societies & Agencies, Cmd. 5499, 1937
Report of the Care of Children Committee (Curtis) Cmd. 6922, 1946.
Report of the Departmental Committee on the Adoption of Children (Hurst) Cmd., 9248, 1954.
Seventh Report of the Work of the Children's Department, Home Office, 1955.
Eighth Report of the Work of the Children's Department, Home Office, 1961.
The Child, the Family, and the Young Offender, Cmd., 2742, 1965.

British and United Nations publications
Robina S. Addis: *Mental Health Aspects of Adoption*, National Association for Mental Health, 1950.
J. Bowlby: *Child Care and the Growth of Love*, Penguin Books, 1951.
J. Bowlby: *Maternal Care and Mental Health*, WHO, 1951.
L. J. Blom-Cooper: 'Historical Development of Legal Adoption', *Child Adoption*, Autumn 1956.
Child Adoption, Quarterly Journal of the Standing Conference of Societies Registered for Adoption.
P. Gray and E. Parr: 'Children in Care and the Recruitment of Foster Parents', Social Survey, 1957.
M. Humphrey and C. Ounsted: 'Adoptive Families Referred for Psychiatric Advice,' *British Journal of Psychiatry*, 109 : 462, 1963.
M. Kornitzer: *Child Adoption in the Modern World*, Putnam, 1952.
National Association for Mental Health: A Survey Based on Adoption Case Records, 1953.
National Institute for Social Work Training and The National Council of Social Service: *A Code of Practice for Research in the Personal Social Services*, 1965.
R. A. Parker: 'The Basis for Research in Adoption', *Case Conference*, September, 1963.
R. A. Parker: *Decision in Child Care*, Allen & Unwin (National Institute for Social Work Training Series), 1966.
Dr L. S. Penrose: 'Heredity as it concerns Adoption', in Standing Conference of Societies Registered for Adoption Report of Residential Conference, 1953.

Jane Rowe: *Yours by Choice*, Mills & Boon, 1959.

Lulie A. Shaw: 'Following up Adoptions', *British Journal of Psychiatric Social Work*, November, 1953.

Standing Conference of Societies Registered for Adoption: 'Adoption Societies' Practice', 1964.

A. M. McWhinnie: A Study of Adoption—The social circumstances & adjustment in adult life of 58 adopted children (presented as Ph.D. Thesis December 1959, Edinburgh University).

United Nations: Department of Social Affairs, *Study on Adoption of Children*, UN Publications, 1953.

World Health Organisation, Technical Report Series No. 70, 'Mental Health Aspects of Adoption', 1953.

M. Yelloly: 'Factors relating to an adoption decision by the mothers of illegitimate infants', *Sociological Review*, Vol. 13, No. 1., March, 1965.

American Publications

American Academy of Pediatrics: *Adoption of Children*, 1960.

R. F. Brenner and R. Michaels: 'A follow-up study of Adoptive Families', Child Adoption Research Committee, Louise Wise Services Inc., 1951.

Donald Brieland: 'An Experimental Study of the Selection of Adoptive Parents at Intake', Child Welfare League of America, 1959.

F. G. Brown: Highlights in Unmarried Mothers' Services and Adoption, Louise Wise Services, Inc., 1955.

F. G. Brown: 'Supervision of the Child in the Adoptive Home', *Child Welfare*, 34 : 1955 (March).

F. G. Brown: 'What do we seek in Adoptive Parents', *Social Casework*, 32 : 155, 1951.

F. G. Brown: *The Use of Group Meetings for Prospective Adoptive Parents*, Louise Wise Services, Inc., 1954.

F. G. Brown: *Adoption of Children with Special Needs*, Child Welfare League of America, 1959.

F. G. Brown: 'Services to Adoptive Parents after Legal Adoption', *Child Welfare*, 38, No. 7, 1959.

Florence G. Brown: *Services to Parents and their Adopted Children in Later Years*, Louise Wise Services, Inc., 1959.

R. Carson: *So you want to adopt a baby*, Public Affairs Pamphlet, 173.

Child Welfare League of America: *Standards for Adoption Service*, 1958.

Child Welfare League of America: *Standards for Services to Unmarried Parents*, 1960.

Children's Bureau, Dept. of Health, Education & Welfare: 'When you Adopt a Child', Folder 13, 1947.

Child Welfare League of America: *Child Welfare as a field of Social Work Practice*.

Child Welfare League of America: *Adoption Practices, Procedures and Problems*, 1949 and 1952.

H. Gordon: *Adoption Practices, Procedures & Problems*, Child Welfare League of America, 1952.

H. David Kirk: 'Nonfecund People as Parents—Some Social and Psychological Considerations', *Fertility & Sterility* 14:3, 1963.

H. David Kirk: Five Lectures on Parent-Child Relationships in Adoption, Whittier College & McGill University, 1961.

H. David Kirk: 'A Dilemma of Adoptive Parenthood', *Marriage & Family Living*, XXI No. 4, 1959.

H. David Kirk: 'The Fate of a Profession's Ameliorative Prescription', McGill University & Whittier College.

H. David Kirk: *Shared Fate: A Theory of Adoption & Mental Health*, Free Press of Glencoe, 1964.

Mignon Krause: *How do we recognise capacities & problems in surrogate parents?*, Louise Wise Services, 1956.

Eda J. Le Shan: *You and Your Adopted Child*, Public Affairs Pamphlet, 274.

L. Raymond: *Adoption and After*, New York, Harper, 1955.

J. H. Reid: 'The Role of the Social Agency in Adoption', *Pediatrics*, 20:369, 1957.

Julius B. Richmond: 'Research in Child Welfare', *Child Welfare*, April 1959.

F. Rondell & R. Michals: *The Adopted Family*, Crown Publications, 1951.

M. Shapiro: *A Study of Adoption Practice*
      Vol. I   Adoption Agencies & the Children they serve
        II   Selected Scientific Papers
       III   Adoption of Children with Special Needs.
      Child Welfare League of America.

H. M. Skeels & I. Harms: 'Children with Inferior Social Histories Their Mental Development in Adoptive Homes,' *Journal of Genetic Psychology* 72:283, 1948.

M. Skodak & H. Skeels: 'A final follow-up study of one hundred adopted children', *Journal of Genetic Psychology*, 75, 1949.

J. R. Wittenborn: *The Placement of Adoptive Children*, Charles C. Thomas, 1957.

INDEX